Toxic World
Who is looking after our kids?

A guide for parents
to protect their children
from environmental chemicals
and other toxic substances

Harold E. Buttram, MD
Richard Piccola, MHA

> Destroy a man's mind, his reasoning ability, his
> imagination, and neither gold, silver, mansions, freedom,
> love, nor anything else will matter to him. This is
> EASILY ACCOMPLISHED, IS BEING ACCOMPLISHED
> by simple means; the creation of disease in his body by
> toxic substances in his food; shattering his nervous system,
> hardening his muscles, and deteriorating his mind--
>
> R. Swinburne Clymer, MD, 1958

Foresight/America Foundation for Preconception Care

Quakertown, Pennsylvania.

Our Toxic World: Who is looking after our kids?
A guide for parents to protect their children from environmental chemicals
and other toxic substances
Harold Buttram, MD & Richard Piccola, MHA

© **1996 Foresight/America Foundation for Preconception Care**
5724 Clymer Rd. Quakertown, Pennsylvania 18951
215-529-9026

*All rights reserved. No part of this book may be reproduced or utilized in
any form or by any means, electronic or mechanical, including
photocopying, recording or by any information storage or retrieval
system, without permission in writing from the Publisher.
Inquiries should be addressed to Permissions Department,
Foresight/America Foundation for Preconception Care.*

Cataloging-in-Publication Data   Library of Congress Catalog Card Number 96-86207

Buttram H, Piccola HR
Our Toxic World: Who is looking after our Children?
A guide for parents to protect their children from environmental chemicals and other toxic substances
   p. cm.
   includes bibliograhic references
   ISBN:0-9653616-0-8
   1. Environmental Health threats to children- popular works 2. Pre-conception care - Popular works   3. Allergy in chilren - Popular works 4. Immune system disorders, childhood- Popular works 5. Childhood behavior disorders - Popular Works 6. Pediatric care - Popular works 7. Pregnancy care -Popular works   I Piccola,HR. II Title.

Printed in the United States of America   First Edition   2 3 4 5 6 7 8 9

Book produced and designed by Torode Design Assoc. Philadelphia

Why every parent should read this book:

Is your child ill?
Read the evidence that these factors may be the underlying causes; by modifying or avoiding them,
bring your child back to health:

- Commercial food processing, increasing use of chemical food additives and inadequate screening for pesticides.
- Toxic environmental chemicals.
- Overuse of antibiotics.
- Overuse or improper use of fluoride.
- Current childhood immunization programs

The most complete discussion
of the impact on children of potential toxic
substances now available to concerned parents

If you are about to begin a family, learn how to conceive the healthiest baby possible.

Here are the studies, conducted by the medical community and the US government, that will show the relationship between the health of your child and the prevalence of environmental poisons. Based on this evidence, this book guides parents in ways to protect their children from the causes of increased health and behavioral problems.

To Nim -

Grandmother to thousands,
guardian angel to all those yet to come.

Nearly fifteen years ago Belinda "Nim" Barnes, a maternity health care worker, decided she had enough with the large petrochemical, pharmaceutical and agricultural industries that were literally poisoning the nation's population with their synthetic drugs, fertilizers, pesticides and food processing additives. Having done her homework well, she gathered scientific data from the United States, England and Europe. Her worst fears were confirmed: adverse birth statistics in the United Kingdom and United States were appallingly on the rise.

Ms. Barnes could not let this sad situation continue; so with the help of a few good friends and the support of her beloved husband, Peter, Foresight was born. The focus of Foresight is a five part health care program which prepares couples for conception.

Armed with her statistics (many from government

publications), she attempted to notify the government, and the chemical and medical establishments. Not only did she have door after door slammed in her face, she found herself under attack. No matter where she turned the large political, medical and industrial establishments did their best to stop her. Thank God for this wife, mother and grandmother who never gave up. With typical "British bulldog determination" and a few very loyal friends, she brought the establishment to its knees and is now personally assisting the organizing of Foresight clinics in the United States and several countries throughout the world.

Disclaimer:

Nothing in this work should be construed
as medical advice.
It is intended purely as a source of information
for patients and families.
For any question concerning medical decisions,
the reader should consult his or her physician.

Contents

Acknowledgments, **1**

Introduction, **3**

1. Preconception care, **9**
2. The case for organic foods, **17**
3. Human studies of food additives & nutrition, **23**
4. Chemical food additives and hyperactivity in children, **27**
5. Volatile organic compounds : contributory causes of learning disabilities and behavior problems in children, **33**
6. The importance of light for the hyperactive child, **51**
7. Water pollution, **53**
8. Toxic heavy metals: lead, cadmium, mercury, antimony and aluminum, **57**

9. Fluoridation: *pros and cons*, **65**

10. Overuse of antibiotics and the need for alternatives, **71**

11. Current childhood vaccination programs: do they cause more disease than they prevent? **81**.

12. Multiple chemical sensitivity: causes, mechanisms, treatment, **97**

13. Combined exposures to multiple chemicals may greatly enhance their toxicity, **105**

14. Food allergies and childhood behavior, **109**

15. Prenatal influences: Effects of the mother's thoughts and emotions on the baby-to-be during pregnancy, **117**

16. Health freedom in America, **127**

17. Conclusions, **129**

Appendix
  I   Case reports of environmental illness, **133**
  II Contaminated school buildings, **149**
  III Preconception Care Program intake forms, **158**

Index, **165**

About the authors, **167**

How to order this book, **168**

Acknowledgments

Ignatius Loyola taught us that the beginning of any prayer is the acknowledgments of all the gifts God has given us. In that spirit I would like to begin this book with thanking some of the people who made it a reality.

Firstly, to Belinda Barnes, who not only encouraged us to write this book but lovingly harassed us until it was completed.

To Victoria Brattini whose help in editing, deciphering my impossible handwriting and using her ever-present mothering instincts kept this book on track.

And to Theron Randolph, MD, who as the Father of Environmental Medicine, influenced a great many physicians and brought to the forefront the profound effects environmental hazards have on health. Dr. Randolph recently passed away.

To our wives, who often suffer from neglect as a result of work schedules which, by their natures, are not always subject to control.

2 *Our toxic world - Who is looking after our kids?*

INTRODUCTION
Who is looking after our kids?

To paraphrase Charles Dickens, these are difficult times, but they are also exciting times. They are dangerous times, but they are also times of unprecedented opportunity.

American children today may be confronted with the greatest difficulty and danger that can be placed on any generation, that of a subtle deterioration in health, largely the result of an increasingly hostile and toxic environment. Considering the circumstances, the marvel is that many do turn out well.

Children are much more vulnerable to toxic exposures than adults. Because they have borne the brunt of these exposures and suffered the consequences in terms of impaired health, it can be predicted that the present generation of children, in years to come, will find definitive answers in terms of restoring a clean human environment and restoring natural balances that all too often, have been disrupted by modern technology.

It has been said that difficulties carry the seeds for their own cure. In the present case, the ultimate cure must rest with the children. It is fairly safe to anticipate that the present generation of children will become the culture bearers of the future.

Increasing health problems in children today largely involve two closely related and interacting systems of the body, the immune system and the brain and nervous system. Health problems involving these systems express themselves as various manifestations of crippled immune systems, delayed development, and "minimal brain dysfunction."

Allergic disorders such as asthma are rapidly increasing, both in frequency and severity.[1,2] Although more difficult to quantify statistically, susceptibility to common viral infections and their complications appears to have increased on a scale largely unknown in earlier generations, as indicated by the increasing numbers of children who are becoming dependent on frequent or prolonged courses of antibiotics.

Corresponding increases have taken place in behavioral disorders, attention deficit hyperactive disorder (ADHD), and learning disabilities. ADHD, with its long-term consequences in terms of impaired learning capacity and social adjustment difficulties that commonly ensue in later adolescence, is arguably one of the foremost health problems of our times.[3,4]

Although statistics confirm the increasing prevalence of ADHD and related problems among children,[5] statistics alone do not tell the entire story. Many factors involved are subtle and intangible and are difficult to measure statistically. Perhaps the best way to gain insight into the pervasiveness of the problem is to talk with veteran teachers with a perspective of 20 or 30 years teaching experience. In our office we have asked a number of these teachers inquiring if they have observed a change in children during their teaching careers. Without exception, they have replied there has been a dramatic change, most notably since the 1970s. Steadily increasing numbers of children, they report, are restless, impulsive, less focused, less able to maintain sustained concentration, and therefore, less able to learn.

Pediatric physician Lendon Smith estimates that 6% to 8% of children are hyperactive in the average elementary school classroom, whereas in the 1950s this problem was rarely seen.

The primary therapy today for ADHD is Ritalin® or related drugs, despite studies showing that the long-term benefits are negligible or at best questionable when used without other therapies.[5,6]

There is a growing consensus that the causes of these adverse health trends among American children can be placed in four categories, which will be the subjects of later chapters:

- Commercial food processing including increasing use of chemical food additives and inadequate screening for pesticide residues.
- Toxic environmental chemicals.
- Overuse of antibiotics.
- Overuse or improper use of fluoride.

To this we feel compelled to add a fifth category:

- Current childhood immunizations - which will take many readers by surprise, as few people today question the efficacy of these vaccines. However, if we are to do justice to today's children, it must be included.

The question is not about the principle of immunization, which is an ongoing natural process, but about the current forms and schedules. When vaccines simulate natural processes, we believe their use can be relatively safe as well as protective, but we do not believe this is the case with current vaccine programs.

There are three basic concerns about current childhood vaccines, which will be reviewed at greater length in another chapter of this book.

The first is that viral vaccines are incubated in animal tissues and, therefore, may carry animal genetic material into the child, setting the stage for later disease.

Second, live virus vaccines are subject to viral contamination.

A third concern, current schedules call for numerous vaccines during the first six months of life of the child, which is certainly a departure from natural processes. Natural infectious challenges, according to standard pediatric texts, come an average of once every 6 weeks following birth, the great majority of which occur without illness. Simultaneous vaccines over a short period of time comprise a wide variant from this natural process. Also, all vaccines, with one exception that is given orally, are injected by needles directly into the system, thereby bypassing the mucosal immune system (the secretory IgA system of the gastrointestinal and respiratory systems) which ordinarily cushion a majority of infectious challenges.

It is difficult to conceive that these abnormal challenges would not use up to an abnormal extent the limited reservoir of the highly immature immune system of the infant, thereby creating long-term and weakening imbalances.

How then can we restore to children that most precious of all gifts, a healthy body with strength, stamina, and a stable nervous system? We believe that meaningful progress will best come about through public education. Large portions of the public are already seeking sound guidance in this area. Above all, there should be freedom of choice in matters pertaining to health. Those seeking health for themselves and their families must return to more natural patterns of living. This requires effort and, very often, the braving of public opinion. This cannot come about in a society where basic freedoms in the health field are denied.

References

1. Weitzman M, et al. Recent trends in the prevalence and severity of asthma. JAMA. 1992;268(19):2673-2677.

2. Hunt LW, et al. Accuracy of the death certificate in a population-based study of asthmatic patients. JAMA. 1993;269(15):1947-1952.

3. Satterfield JH, et al. Therapeutic interventions to prevent delinquency in hyperactive boys. J Am Acad Child Adolesc Psychiatry. 1987;26(1):56-64.

4. Barkley RA, et al. The adolescent outcome of hyperactive children diagnosed by research criteria: I. An 8-year prospective follow-up study. J Am Acad Child Adolesc Psychiatry. 1990;29(4):546-557.

5. Wolraich ML, et al. Stimulant medication use by primary care physicians in the treatment of attention deficit hyperactivity disorder. Pediatrics. 1990;86:95-101.

6. Hechtman L. Adolescent outcome of hyperactive children treated with stimulants in childhood: a review. Psychopharmocol Bull. 1985;21:178.

Chapter 1
Preconception care

"Start at the beginning," "as you sow, so shall you reap," "planning makes it happen," and "your future is directly dependent on your ability to think clearly, concentrate and stay on track." These are clichés we've all heard but rarely thought about when planning to have children. When applied to our children's health, they translate into two very powerful words: preconception care.

The Preconception Care Program, developed by the Foresight Foundation, is an organized program that identifies and reduces reproductive risks before conception and prepares both parents for the pregnancy. Its goal is to ensure that prior to conception, a woman and her partner are both healthy and practicing lifestyle behaviors with the aim of having a healthy baby.

We need a preconception care program for a number of reasons. Consider that according to the Center for Disease Control, the United States ranked 23rd on the International Ranking for Infant Mortality in 1991. For every 1,000 live births, there are 9.8 infant deaths before age one. During the past five years little has changed to improve those statistics. This nation has one of the highest infant mortality rates in the world. The miracle of modern technology has allowed us to save some very sick children but it has not improved the quality of life for many of them and in some instances it has only guaranteed a lifetime of health problems. We have not perfected having healthy babies but we perfected the technology for helping babies that would have died.

Low birth weight for gestational age affects one in 15 babies and has been implicated in failure-to-thrive babies. Eleven percent of our babies are born prematurely and according to Iams, Johnson and Creasey (*Clinical Obstetrics & Gynecology Journal*, 1988) more than 75% of perinatal mortality and morbidity in infants without congenital anomalies are caused by complications of prematurity.

Consider also that hospitalization costs for low birth weight infants in the United States. ranges from $16,136 to $174,278 compared to $2,923 for initial hospital costs of a normal weight baby. The figures were supplied by the March of Dimes.

The March of Dimes states that 30 to 40 percent of birth defects are linked to known medical, genetic, environmental and psychosocial factors that can be, to some degree, prevented.

In 1989 Congress passed a law which designated the '90s as "The Decade of the Brain."[1] The text begins: "Whereas it is estimated that 50 million Americans are affected each year by disorders and disabilities that involve the brain." The law then lists such disorders and disabilities, including those "resulting for prenatal events" and continues with: "Whereas it is estimated that treatment, rehabilitation and related costs represent a total economic burden of 305 billion annually." The law ends by stating: "The president is authorized and requested to issue a proclamation calling on public and private institutions as well as the people of the United States to observe the decade with appropriate programs and activities."

Congress also published a 360 page report on neurotoxicity which documents the grounds for this legislation emphasizing treatment and prevention.[2] It is interesting to note that a survey of individuals in whom long-term disabilities originated prior to age 18 and were receiving Social Security showed that in 75% percent of the cases the defect had its origin *before birth*. Disabilities included cerebral palsy, mental retardation, epilepsy, visual and auditory impediments, disorders of speech and poor school performance.

It is also estimated that roughly 40% of all pregnancies in the United States are unplanned. Those that are planned actually start preparation for a healthy baby after conception has already taken place. In the biological sense the life process, and the hazard to development of the life process, begins about 100 days before conception, when both the male and female germ cells (sperm and egg) begin their maturation process. It is at this time that both the sperm and the egg are most vulnerable to toxins, nutritional deficiencies and radiation.

The answer to all these difficulties lies in changing one little word: *"unplanned."* We must plan for healthy babies, and we must begin before conception occurs.

Fast, effective and inexpensive, The Preconception Care program is the ultimate risk management program for prospective parents who want to do all they can to insure a healthy baby.

The program has five basic components. Ideally it begins four to six months before conceiving. This enables time for tests to be completed and evaluated, and for both potential parents to optimize their own health.

Parents first meet with a Preconception Care counselor who assists with filling out forms. (See index)

After reviewing these intake forms with the patients, the doctor will do a general physical examination of each potential parent, including a battery of routine tests designed to determine general health, nutrient levels, and for Chlamydia, a silent venereal disease prevalent in men and women that can be contracted without sexual contact.

An integral part of The Preconception Care Program is the inclusion of environmental medicine. This field of medicine recognizes that our increasingly polluted environment is a major source of chronic illness and quiet cellular damage. These illnesses include reaction to well-known chemicals and to many seemingly harmless chemicals that are used in our homes, offices and workplaces. They are manifested as mental, emotional, and physical problems that range from headaches and depression to multiple muscle and joint aches and pains.

The Preconception Care's Environmental Program includes the detection of food sensitivities, allergies, and chemical sensitivities in both parents. Psychosocial substances such as caffeine, nicotine and recreational drugs are also discussed.

Nutrition counseling is an important component of the Program. Good nutrition is vitally important to all stages of life, especially before conception occurs. While those in medical science are aware of the consequences brought on by a profound state of malnutrition, we are only beginning to understand the potential impact of more subtle nutritional deficiencies on pregnancy. However, the evidence continues to build for a role in Preconception Care. On September 14, 1992, the United States Public Health Service recommended that all women of childbearing age take extra folic acid, a B-vitamin, to prevent neural tube defects (NTD) that effect one to two of every 1,000 babies born each year. It is not enough to tell women to take the vitamin after they are pregnant because the birth defects occur when the fetus's spinal column is fusing, at about two weeks after the first missed menstrual period. Many women are still unaware they are pregnant at that time.

Fathers also must be nutritionally aware. The journal, *Proceedings of the Natural Academy of Science* (February 1992) published a study which demonstrated a direct relationship between a diet low in vitamin C and increased DNA damage in sperm cells. The consequences include infertility and decreased sperm function in perspective fathers and some birth defects and cancers in their offspring.

Nutritional deficiencies such as those mentioned above can have such a dramatic effect on the health of our children. There are other subtle nutritional deficiencies with equally high damaging impacts on pregnancy and birth.

The Preconception Care program looks closely at the diet of both prospective parents. Recommendations are tailored to each couple's lifestyle and ethnic heritage. Depending on their dietary history, and the blood and hair test results, supplementation may be advised. The Program is based on the assumption that the best insurance for obtaining all the essential nutrients is to eat a wide variety of fresh, colorful, organically grown food. To meet that goal, patients are guided in how to choose and prepare food and how to measure a serving size. They are further educated to know what nutrients are supplied by which foods and the function of those nutrients in the role of having a healthy baby.

The genetics portion of the Preconception Care Program provides couples with a family "pedigree." Knowledge of a couple's risk can be found by taking a complete family history which should include inquiring about previous occurrences in the family of mental retardation, birth defects, known genetic diseases, early death and chronic health problems in the first, second and third degree relatives of the couple in questions.

Such issues as ethnicity and consanguinity should also be addressed. That knowledge would best be acquired *prior* to that person's having children in hope of enabling those individuals who are at risk for having children with serious illnesses to make well informed decisions about their family planning. To this end, genetic counseling is an irreplaceable component of a program in preconception care.

Since it is important that the couple avoid pregnancy until they have reached optimal health, appropriate family planning is essential. The timing of ovulation is a critical factor in the conception process. Prospective parents are taught the sympto-thermal method of fertility awareness which combines observations of cervical placement, cervical mucus, and basal body temperature. Books, films and individual counseling help parents to understand this method.

The knowledge that your baby's health was included in your family planning is but one of the benefits of The Preconception Care Program, and knowing that you did everything possible to have a healthy baby provides you with great peace of mind.

For more information about Preconception Care write to:

>   *Foresight-America Foundation*
>   *5724 Clymer Road*
>   *Quakertown, PA 18951*
>   *Phone:* 1(800)-Let-Heal

References:

1. 101 USC §58.

2. *Neurotoxicity: Identifying and Controlling Poisons of the Nervous System.* Washington, DC: US Congress, Office of Technology Assessment; 1990

Chapter 2
The case for organic foods

During an interview with a young woman who was raised in Iran and later immigrated to the United States, the topic of nutrition was discussed. She commented that she missed the fruits grown in Iran, which were tasty and luscious. In comparison fruits grown in the United States were flat and relatively tasteless, often leaving her dissatisfied. This simple anecdote strikes at the heart of the differences between organically grown foods and those grown with chemical fertilizers, pesticides, and herbicides.

In 1992, there was a cable television program hosted by David Suzuki entitled, "Down on the Farm." The scene was a wheat farming area in western Canada. In the course of the program soil from one farm devoted to organic farming was compared with soil of an adjacent farm using chemical methods. The differences were evident. Soil from the organic farm was darker and more porous, and it crumbled easily when handled. Soil from the adjacent farm, in contrast, had a putty-like stickiness.

How did the organic farmer compare financially with his neighbors? In good years, they came out about the same, but in years with adverse weather conditions, the organic farmer did "dramatically better." He went on to say that in the earlier years he had been the object of quite a bit of good-natured kidding by his neighbors for his antiquated methods. "They aren't kidding any more," he said smilingly.

The methods used by the organic farmer were those still used in many other countries: crop rotations with a combination of manure and periodic plowing under of crops, thus maintaining the topsoil in a rich and fertile condition.

Another aspect explaining the differences was that, by using pesticides and herbicides, the chemical farmers tended to kill out worms and microorganisms native to the soil. This reduces the porosity of the soil and its capacity to hold moisture. It also reduces the transformation of inorganic minerals into a colloidal state in which minerals are much more readily taken up by the plants.

The superiority of organic foods versus supermarket foods was documented by Bob L. Smith with Doctor's Data of West Chicago.[1] In the study, dry ashed concentrates of foods were analyzed for mineral content on state-of-the-art instruments. The average elemental concentration of nutrient minerals in organic foods on a fresh weight basis was found to be about twice that of commercial foods. Also the average content of the toxic metals, aluminum, cadmium, and mercury was lower in the organic foods.

Pesticide residues in foods are of growing concern to health authorities. In 1989, a report sponsored by the Natural Resources Defense Council, Washington DC, estimated that at least 17% of preschool children (3 million American children at the time) were exposed to neurotoxic pesticides from fruits and vegetables alone at levels far above those described as safe by the federal government.[2] In *Pesticides in Diets of Infants and Children*,[3] a book was sponsored by the National Research Council and National Academy of Sciences, the inadequacies of present screening systems for pesticide residues in foods were painstakingly reviewed.

Although chlorinated pesticides such as DDT and chlordane have been banned from use in the United States, they still find their way to the American consumer through imported foods, largely from Third World countries where there are no bans on their use. It has been estimated that 40% of produce in the American marketplace is imported during winters.

Solutions for consumers:

In planning diets for families with children or who are planning on having children in the future, special emphasis should be placed on obtaining organic fruits and fruit juices. Children consume far more of these foods than adults, and fruits are more likely to be contaminated with pesticides than other classes of foods.[2]

Educated consumers can accelerate a change to safer foods through their power in the marketplace, by creating a greater demand for organically grown fruits and vegetables, thus providing an incentive for farmers to decrease their use of pesticides.

Unfortunately, organic foods are more expensive, and a total organic food diet is beyond the financial capacity of many young couples. As an alternative, the couple could plant their own vegetable garden using proven organic methods. Another alternative is to wash all vegetables and fruits, soaking them in a pan with a little added vinegar or baking soda followed by thorough rinsing. Vegetables and fruits should be peeled when appropriate (apples, pears, etc). Potatoes and carrots should be scrubbed with a vegetable scrub brush. Outer leaves of cabbage and lettuce, and celery should be trimmed. These measures will go far toward reducing pesticide levels.

Comments on contemporary eating patterns:

Senior citizens of today will recall how in earlier times there was a basic pattern of prepared family meals. These were generally unhurried and conducive to relaxation and enjoyment. The fare consisted of plain, simple, staple foods. Chemical additives were very limited in comparison with today's standards. "Treats" were limited to special occasions.

Under today's conditions for young couples,

where both must often be wage earners in order to make ends meet, this pattern often falls by the wayside. Commercially prepared "fast foods" are increasingly becoming the norm. In addition to having chemical additives, they are almost invariably nutritionally inferior to unprocessed foods.

With the very high rate of broken families today, one must wonder if the decline of the family meal and its attendant family bonding is playing a role.

Young couples, should try to set priorities in which this institution is held at or near the top in spite of duresses and time pressures of daily living. We should all remember the foods our grandparents ate and return to the pattern of plain, simple foods. Although the diets of former generations were not always ideal, nine times out of ten they were vastly superior to the average fare of today.

Conclusions:

Balanced nutrition is one of the basic cornerstones of health, prolonged youthfulness, adequate energy for accomplishing one's goals in life, and a resistant immune system. It also goes far in protecting against toxic chemical exposures.

References

1. Smith BL. Organic foods vs supermarket foods: element levels. J Appl Nutr 1993;45(1):35-39. Reprints available from: Doctor's Data, Inc., PO Box 111 West Chicago, IL 60185-9986.

2. Intolerable Risk: Pesticides in Our Children's Foods. Washington, DC: Natural Resources Defense Council; 1989.

3. Pesticides in Diets of Infants and Children. Washington, DC: National Research Council and National Academy of Sciences, National Academy Press;.1993.

Recommended reading and viewing

Bradley FM, ed. Rodale's Chemical-Free Yard and Garden. Emmaus, PA: Rodale Press; 1991.

Galland L, Buchman DD. Superimmunity of Kids. New York: Dell Publishing; 1988.

Gislason SJ. Core Diet for Kids. Vancouver, BC: Persona Audiovisual Productions;1989.

Matsen J. Eating Alive. Blaine, WA: N.D. Crompton Books, Ltd; 1987.

Reed B, Knickelbine S, Knickelbine M. Food, Teens & Behavior. Manitowoc, WI: Natural Press; 1983.

Rodale's All-New Encyclopedia of Organic Gardening. Emmaus, PA: Rodale Press

Rodale's Chemical-Free Yard and Garden. Emmaus PA: Rodale Press; 1991.

CHAPTER 3

Human studies on food additives and nutrition

The elimination of foods with chemical additives and the substitution of unprocessed foods with higher nutritive values can have a profoundly beneficial effect on childhood and adolescent behavioral patterns. It also results insignificant improvement in scholastic performance. The truth of these statements has been demonstrated in a series of studies in schools and juvenile correction institutions.[1-4]

There were two phases to the studies.Phase one involved the lowering of sugar and the elimination of foods with artificial colors and flavors and the preservatives, BHA and BHT, in the school cafeterias of 803 New York public schools from 1978 to 1983.

The changes did not involve any increase in cafeteria budgets. The candy in vending machines was replaced with such things as fruit, popcorn, and peanuts. During the study, there was a 15.7% increase in academic rankings of students in these schools above the rest of the nation's schools which used the same standardized test. Before this 15.7% gain, the annual change in national ratings had not exceeded 1%.

The second phase introduced the same dietary policies into 12 juvenile correctional institutions located in different parts of the nation. In every instance, this change was followed by an average of 47% reduction in violence and other forms of antisocial behavior. The following table lists the changes that were made in the menus:

**Permanent implemented changes
in the Virginia and Alabama Diet Behavior Programs
designed to control the consumption of
low nutrient density (high sugar/fat) foods**

1. Breakfast cereals with added sugars were replaced with cereals that were not presweetened.
2. Canned fruits packed in syrup were rinsed in cold water before being served.
3. Kool-Aid® and soft drinks were replaced with a variety of fruit juices - orange, tomato, V-8,® grapefruit, apple and grape.
4. Iced tea was served unsweetened.
5. Soft drink machines were replaced with fruit juice machines.
6. Table sugar was replaced with honey. (People tend to use a little less sugar when sweetening their food with honey rather than sucrose).

7. Refined white breads were replaced with whole wheat breads.
8. White rice was replaced with brown rice.
9. Processed foods were replaced with fresh produce when available at similar prices.
10. Snack foods high in sugar and fat were replaced with other foods. Candy bars, ice cream, cookies and refined carbohydrate snacks - pastries, potato chips, etc. - were no longer allowed. They were replaced with fresh fruits, fresh vegetables and a variety of nuts, cheeses, fruit juices and whole grain crackers.
11. The parents of each juvenile were requested for health reasons to refrain from sending their children foods that contained large amounts of sugar such as candy and pastries.

    The key to successful control of marginally nutritious foods lies in the availability of a large variety of more nutritious alternatives which will be accepted just as readily. Accordingly, the original policy restrictions on selected high-sugar dessert foods and condiments - cake with icing, jelly, etc. - were modified to allow low quantities in most institutions.

References

1. Schoenthaler SJ, et al. The impact of a low food-additive and sucrose diet on academic performance in 803 New York City public schools. *Intern J Biosocial Research.* 1986;8(2):185-195.

2. Schoenthaler SJ. Institutional nutritional policies and criminal behavior. *Nutrition Today.* May/June 1985:16-37.

3. Schoenthaler SJ. Diet and criminal behavior: a criminological evaluation of the Arlington, Virginia proceedings. *Intern J Biosocial Research.* 1987;9(2):161-181.

4. Schoenthaler SJ. Brains and vitamins. *Lancet.* 1991;337:728-729. Letters to the Editor.

CHAPTER 4

Chemical food additives and hyperactivity in children

The increasing pervasiveness of hyperactivity, attention deficit, and related childhood disorders in the United States has been reviewed in the Introduction. Along with toxic environmental chemicals, chemical food additives may be a major contributor to these states in increasing numbers of our children. Russell L. Blaylock, MD, a neurosurgeon, in his book entitled, Excitotoxins, the Taste that Kills,[1] extensively reviews compelling evidence that certain food additives such as monosodium glutamate (MSG) and the sweetener, aspartame, act as excitotoxins that assault the brain and lead to numerous health problems.

The background of MSG, which might be used as a prototype of chemical excitotoxins, is a fascinating one. It was originally developed in Japan as a flavor enhancer for foods. In 1948 a meeting was held at which most of the major food manufacturing giants in America were in attendance. It was concluded that

27

this Japanese flavor-enhancer did have some remarkable properties. Since that time, the American food industry has drastically increased the amount of MSG added to prepared foods, which has doubled every decade since the 1940s. Today MSG is added to most soups, fast foods, chips, frozen foods, ready-made dinners, and canned goods.²

The first indications of problems came in 1957 when two ophthalmology residents tested MSG and aspartate on infant and adult mice while studying a particular eye disorder. What they found came as a complete surprise. After sacrificing the animals and examining tissues under a microscope, they found that in animals tested with MSG, nerve cells in the inner layers of the retinas had been destroyed. The worst damage occurred in newborns, but even adults showed significant injury. They also found similar though less severe damage from aspartate, one of the main ingredients in Nutrasweet,® the artificial sweetener. In 1968, Dr. John Olney, a neuroscientist at Washington University, St. Louis, repeated the same experiment and found that not only did MSG cause severe damage to retinal neurons of the eye, but that it also caused widespread destruction to the hypothalamus and other areas of the brain. Despite the fact that these findings were confirmed in a number of animal experiments with a wide variety of species, few paid attention to this critical discovery. Without a public or professional outcry, the food industry continued adding more and more MSG to foods. Even baby foods contained relatively large doses of MSG.

As explained by Dr. Blaylock, both glutamate and aspartate are neurotransmitters found normally in the brain and spinal cord. (Neurotransmitters are chemical substances released from the terminal ends of nerve cells (axons), which seep through the tiny clefts (synapses) between nerves, attach themselves to the next nerve in line and cause it to fire). Although glutamate and aspartate are two of the most common transmitters in the brain, when their concentrations rise above a critical level, they may become "deadly toxins" by inducing a chain reaction of uncontrolled repetitive firing of nerve cells. This, in turn, depletes energy stores, the end result being death of the nerve cell from exhaustion.

Because abnormally high body levels of MSG and/or aspartame may result in a continual state of hyperexcitability as well as brain injury, Blaylock proposes that exposure to the fetus during pregnancy and the child following birth, may result in learning disabilities, hyperactivity, impaired social judgment, autism, and possibly schizophrenia.

Experiments have demonstrated that early exposure to excitotoxins can result in later behavioral changes and learning impairment. In a carefully controlled study, 22 rats were given low daily doses of MSG for 11 days after birth. The rats exhibited hyperactivity, and they had considerable difficulty in escaping even the simplest mazes, as compared with controls not given MSG. They had difficulty in distinguishing between different types of stimuli and behaved "like animals with lower intelligence."

Additional adverse symptoms and health problems attributed to consumption of foods with MSG include migraine headaches, stomach aches, depression, and asthma.[2]

In the past, MSG was frequently labeled (more properly mislabeled) as hydrolyzed protein, natural flavorings, Chinese seasoning, and a variety of other aliases. Presumably this mislabeling will be corrected by the new law.

Other additives implicated in childhood hyperactivity include artificial food colorings (red and yellow dyes) and artificial flavors. The first and still most widely known person to report that these additives may trigger behavioral and hyperactive reactions was Dr. Ben Feingold, at one time chief of Allergy at the Kaiser-Permanente Medical Center in San Francisco.[3] Although other researchers had difficulty in duplicating Feingold's favorable results, Egger's classic study, which implicated food allergies as a prime factor in the hyperkinetic syndrome, found that food additives and colorants were the most common substances that produced abnormal behavior in the patients.[4] These artificial dyes have also been implicated in allergic reactions.

Several other additives, although not involved in hyperactivity, are of concern: nitrites, sulfites, and the antioxidants butylated hydroxytoluene (BHT) and butylated hydroxyanisole (BHA).

Nitrites are used to cure bacon and other pork products. They protect the consumer from botulism, but unfortunately, nitrites convert to the potent carcinogen, nitrosamine, in the body. This process may be inhibited by adding such antioxidants as ascorbate (vitamin C).

Sulfites are a class of chemicals that can keep cut fruits and vegetables looking fresh, even when they are not. Reactions occur mostly in patients with asthma. their use was largely, unrestricted until 1985 when the United States Food and Drug Administration (FDA) placed a ban on their use in most fresh fruits and vegetables. However, the ban does not cover grapes, fresh-cut potatoes, dried fruits, or wine.

BHT *and* BHA delay rancidity in food products containing fats or oils. They are used in products such as baking mixtures, cereals, instant potatoes, ice cream, candy, chewing gum, gelatin desserts, soup bases, dry mixes for desserts, and other commercially prepared foods. They are suspected of being carcinogenic, and they may cause allergies.

In conclusion, food additives may in some instances serve a useful and necessary purpose, as in the prevention of botulism and other diseases. However, in the early part of this century up until World War II, food additives as we now know them largely did not exist. In those days there was far less sickness among children than today.[5] Is there a connection? We believe that there is!

References

1. Blaylock RL. *Excitotoxins, The Taste That Kills.* Santa Fe, NM:Health Press; 1994.

2. Schwartz GR. *In Bad Taste, The MSG Syndrome,* Santa Fe, NM:Health Press;1988.

3. Feingold B; Miller IN, ed. *Nutrition and Behavior.* Philadelphia: Pa: Franklin Institute Press; 1981. Chap 18.

4. Egger J, et al. Controlled trial of oligoantigenic treatment in the hyperkinetic syndrome. *Lancet;* 1985;540-545.

5. Beasley JD, Swift JJ. *The Kellogg Report; The Impact of Nutrition, Environment and Lifestyle on the Health of Americans.* Anandale-on-Hudson, NY: Institute of Health and Policy Practice, Bard College Center. 1989

Recommended reading

Jacobson MF, Lefferts LY, Garland AW. *Safe Food: Eating Wisely in a Risky World.* Los Angeles,Ca: Living Plant Press; 1991.

Millichap JG. *Environmental Poisons in Our Food.* Chicago, Ill: PNB Publishing; 1993.

Roberts HJ. *Aspartame, (NutraSweet®), Is It Safe?* Philadelphia, Pa: Charles Press; 1990.

Winter R. *Consumer's Dictionary of Food Additives.* New York, NY: Crown Publishers;1989.

CHAPTER 5
Volatile organic compounds: contributory causes of learning disabilities and behavioral problems in children

Volatile organic compounds (VOCs) are a very large class of commercial chemicals that tend to evaporate into and contaminate indoor air of buildings. They enter the human system not only by inhalation, but also through skin absorption.

From the standpoint of human health and welfare, VOCs all share one important characteristic: they are all fat or lipid soluble, and therefore they have an affinity for the fatty or lipid tissues of the body. The brain is a prime target of the VOCs due to its high lipid content and rich blood supply.

Health problems from VOC exposures have largely taken place since World War II. Before World War II, US production of synthetic organic compounds totaled fewer than one billion pounds per year, but by 1976 production had soared to 163 billion pounds per year.[1]

About 70,000 chemicals are used in commerce, of which several hundred are known to be neurotoxic.

However, except for pharmaceuticals, less than 10% have had any testing at all for neurotoxicity, and only a handful of these have been evaluated thoroughly.[2]

The pervasiveness of these chemicals was reflected in a study that showed that 10 volatile chemicals were commonly found in indoor air, drinking water, and exhaled breaths of 400 residents of New Jersey, North Carolina, and North Dakota.[3]

Because the brain is the primary target of VOCs, symptoms are primarily cerebral in nature. Acute symptoms include dizziness, forgetfulness, headaches, mental fogginess, difficulty concentrating, and poor coordination. One of the centers investigating chronic effects of organic solvent exposures is at the University of Pittsburgh where Lisa Morrow, PhD and coworkers have published a series of studies on the effects of solvents on occupationally exposed subjects.[4-10] These findings included social alienation, poor concentration, anxiety, and impairments in learning and memory.

VOC exposure is taking a heavy toll among adults, but the effects may be even greater among our children. It has been estimated that children may be up to 10 times more vulnerable to chemical toxins than adults because of their rapidly growing tissues and organs and the relative immaturity of their detoxification systems.[11]

It is more than coincidental that the present epidemic of hyperactivity and behavioral problems among school children has coincided with steadily increasing levels of VOCs found in modern buildings. Standard neurotoxicology texts point out that behavioral problems may be the earliest sign of chemical toxicity.[12, 13]

In an investigation of three sick building syndrome (SBS) outbreaks, which included two high schools, it was concluded that the chronic fatigue syndrome (CFS) is often associated with SBS. Chronic fatigue immune deficiency syndrome is a condition characterized by overwhelming fatigue, muscle aches, inability to concentrate and other symptoms affecting predominantly young adults.[14]

Respiratory and neurologic symptoms often overlapped with CFS. Symptoms included headaches, fatigue, muscle pains, rhinitis, sinusitis, memory problems, fatigue, low-grade fevers, eye irritation and tearing, and light sensitivity. The authors suggest that the cause may be low levels of contaminants acting "in concert" or synergistically to produce overlapping syndromes. The study was sponsored by Georgetown University Medical Center and the National Institutes of Health.[14]

In the booklet, *Environmental Hazards In Your Schools*, published by the United States Environmental Protection Agency (EPA),[15] it was pointed out that high energy costs encourage the development of tight buildings with poor ventilation. These conditions, combined with the proliferation of indoor contaminants - synthetic materials, cleaning agents, pesticides, printing and copying devices, combustion appliances, tobacco products, and other sources - reduce the quality of indoor air environments and consequently, the health of building occupants.

In the 1970s and 80s, EPA conducted studies which disclosed that important contaminants were often two to five times higher indoors than outdoors. Health problems from indoor air contamination may include fatigue, lethargy, difficulty with concentration, problems with recent memory, hyperactivity in children, and eye/ear/nose/throat irritations.

There is growing public concern about possible adverse effects of toxic environmental chemical exposures on human health, especially that of children. Irene Ruth Wilkenfeld, a retired school teacher with many years of teaching experience, has warned of a relationship between environmental chemicals and the increasing incidence of learning disabilities in children:[16]

> Generations of reformers have tried to revitalize our educational system. To date, the outcome has been disappointing. I strongly believe that one key variable has been overlooked. Virtually no attention has been focused on the environmental school factors that may trigger hypersensitivity reactions and adversely impact a child's ability to learn.
>
> Environmentalists, who have fought to protect nearly every species in the animal kingdom, have overlooked a prime endangered species: our school-aged children. And until school-based

environmental insults are substantially curtailed, our nation's youngsters will continue to fall short of our educational goals.

When parents are provided with instructions and guidelines, it is relatively easy and inexpensive to clean up the home environment and reduce chemical exposures in most instances . For children who are being made ill by chemical exposures, major obstacles to restoration of health often come from their attending schools where they are subjected to heavy chemical exposures.

Wilkenfeld, wrote further on the subject:[17]

> The building and renovation boom in school systems across the country is backfiring in widespread outbreaks of building-associated illnesses, known as the sick school syndrome.
>
> The construction and renovation process can involve significant environmental exposures. If materials are indiscriminately chosen or if the structure is haphazardly designed, the schoolhouse can become a long-term source of chemical contamination.
>
> Indoor air quality in many modern, energy-efficient, "tight" schools is deplorable. Walking into the typical school today is like sealing your head in a ziplock plastic bag filled with noxious fumes. It's like swimming in a toxic terrarium filled with a chemical soup concocted with synthetic construction materials.
>
> We've mistakenly assumed that carpeting, paints, adhesives, sealants, roofing materials and insulation are inert. That is not so. These

synthetically derived products "outgas"- exude a host of volatile organic chemicals into the air. These subliminal stressors are capable of triggering a cascade of devastating symptoms that adversely affect health, mood and behavior, and are thereby capable of undermining academic performance and productivity. Not surprisingly, many chemically injured patients attribute the onset of their illness to renovation and/or construction at home, at school or in the workplace.

The World Health Organization estimates that about 30 percent of US. schools have indoor air quality problems. This figure may be even higher for newly constructed or remodeled facilities.

This is especially significant when we realize the impact on young people. The health risks from air pollution are as much as six times greater for children than for adults, according to Robert Phalem, director of the University of California at Irvine Air Pollution Health Effects Laboratory.

There is mounting evidence that children exposed to classroom contaminants do not live up to their full academic potential.

VOCs can be assigned to three major categories: pesticides, solvents and other volatile chemicals, and formaldehyde.

Pesticides

In the 1960s and 70s, the use of chlorinated pesticides, such as DDT, Dieldrin, and Chlordane, was banned from use in the United States due to their persistence in the environment and the human body. Since that time, organophosphate pesticides have become the most commonly used class of pesticides in the United States.

The organophosphates are designed to poison the nervous systems of unwanted pests. They are related to the nerve gasses of chemical warfare.

Children may be subjected to continual or repeated exposures to organophosphate pesticides through pesticide residues in fruits and vegetables and through their use in or about school buildings and homes.

There are very good reasons for concern about repeated exposures of children to pesticides, even at low doses.

- Numerous epidemiologic studies of adults with occupational exposures to organophosphate pesticides have shown evidence of neurologic damage manifested by subtle personality changes and learning disabilities.[18-29] These changes may take place in the absence of any signs of acute illness.

- It has been estimated that children may be up to 10 times more vulnerable to chemical toxicities than adults [11]

- Pesticides are lipid soluble, just like other VOCs. The brain is a primary target because of its rich blood supply and high proportion of lipids.

- Organophosphates may persist in indoor air up to 21 days following indoor application, according to William Forbes, Pest Control Manager of the Montgomery County, Maryland School District.

- The EPA has not required testing of pesticides for delayed neurotoxicity.[30]

- The present standard test for organophosphate toxicity (red blood cell cholinesterase) is relatively insensitive. In some instances neurologic damage may take place without abnormalities in this test.[31, 32]

In closing this section on pesticides, a number of school districts throughout the country are adopting "Integrated Pest Management," which involves the control of pests without chemicals. These measures are proving to be effective, and less expensive than pesticides.

Organic solvents and other volatile chemicals:

As previously reviewed, organic solvents are lipid-soluble chemicals that have an affinity for the fatty tissues of the body. The most common symptoms from exposures are cerebral in nature and include dizziness, headaches, drowsiness, mental fogginess, inability to concentrate, memory lapses, irritability, anxiety, and mood changes. Chronic occupational exposures in adults are known to bring about memory and learning impairments and adverse personality changes.[4-10]

Common indoor sources of organic solvent exposure are paints, varnishes, waxes, sealants, glues, carpets, paint strippers, wood preservatives, aerosol sprays, cleaning solutions and disinfectants, air fresheners, personal cosmetics, and stored fuels. In schools, art classes and hobby shops may be sources of significant exposures. Leaky or poorly ventilated oil or gas heating units may result in petrochemical fumes in the air.

Although improvements are beginning to come about, many commercial carpets made from synthetic materials pose a special problem. A story is told about EPA headquarters in Washington DC. This building, completed a few years ago according to the most modern specifications, proved to be a major embarrassment to the EPA, especially considering that it is the primary responsibility of this agency to protect the public from harmful exposures. Soon after occupancy of the new building, a large proportion of employees became ill. The source of these illnesses proved to be the combination of a defective ventilation system and outgassing of toxic chemicals from new wall-to-wall carpets.

Synthetic carpets may be the source of a variety of outgassing chemicals including 4-phenylcyclohexane (4-PCH), formaldehyde, styrene, vinyl acetate, isooctane and styrene butadiene.[33]

Styrene butadiene, a byproduct from latex backing used in many carpets, has been found to cause a significant increase in malignant tumors in animals.

In an epidemiologic study of 8017 males with occupational exposures to butadiene involved in latex manufacture, it was found that there was increased incidence of lymphatic cancers and leukemias.[34,35]

Formaldehyde:

In her doctoral thesis, "*The Psychological and Educational Implications of Formaldehyde Toxicology,*" Joan Swanson stated,

> Formaldehyde exposure should be considered when teachers observe one or more of the following: Marked increase in absenteeism, tiredness, changes in functioning levels, spotty learning, significant drop in grades, and emotional instability.[36]

Primary sources of airborne formaldehyde in buildings may include particle board subflooring and paneling, plywood paneling, urea formaldehyde foam insulation in older buildings (this form of insulation was phased out in the early 1980s), paints, waxes, glues, upholstery and drapery fabrics, cabinets and other classroom furniture made from particle board. It may also be present in newsprint, permanent-pressed clothes, incomplete combustion of petrochemical fuels, cigarette smoke, and carbonless copying paper.

In addition to impairments of mental function, formaldehyde causes irritations of eyes, throat, and respiratory system. Concentrations above 0.5 to 1.0

ppm may be detected by odor. Concentrations above 0.3 ppm may cause increased airway resistance in breathing and therefore may aggravate asthma.

Conclusions:

Hyperactivity and behavioral problems are epidemic in today's schools. Irrational, wanton crime has become a leading social problem among juveniles in American cities.

Perhaps one of the most urgent questions confronting modern society is whether toxic chemical exposures are capable of bringing about these adverse personality and behavioral changes among our youngsters. If this is indeed the case, then reducing these toxic exposures should become of urgent importance, second to none.

The following anecdotal report vividly exemplifies the potential of toxic chemicals to bring about Jekyll/Hyde personality changes. Although somewhat comical in itself, it carries serious overtones for modern society.

As reported in *Psychosomatics*,[37] a professor of medicine at a New England university applied a tick powder daily to his male cat during a summer month. Within 10 days after starting the applications, large numbers of dead or injured mice and birds were noted on the front lawn. The cat brought additional birds and mice into the house where he frequently attacked them with claws and teeth. Such behavior by a previously docile cat bewildered the professor and caused him to remark, "my cat has become a murderer."

There were at the same time personality changes in the professor. Although he wore gloves during applications of the tick powder, he would often breathe the dust as it escaped into the air. The professor's housemate became alarmed by the increasing aggressiveness and "continual rage" of the professor. Because of distinct fear of physical attack by the professor, the companion left the premises. It was at this point that the professor and his companion independently realized that the tick powder could have been the cause of these changes, and its use was terminated. Within one week aggressive behavior ceased in both cat and man.

References

1. *Multiple Chemical Sensitivities*. Washington DC: National Research Council, National Academy Press; 1989:52.

2. *Multiple Chemical Sensitivities*. Washington DC: National Research Council, National Academy Press; 1989:2.

3. Wallace LA, et al.The TEAM study: personal exposures to toxic substances in air, drinking water, and breath of 400 residents of New Jersey, North Carolina and North Dakota. *Environ Res*.1987;43:290-307

4. Morrow LA, et al. PET and neurobehavioral evidence of tetrabromoethane encephalopathy. J *Neuropsych*; 1990;2:431-435.

5 Morrow LA, et al. Cacosmia and neurobehavioral dysfunction associated with occupational exposure to mixtures of organic solvents. AmJ *Psychiatry*. 1988;145:1442-1445

6. Ryan CMM, et al. Assessment of neuropsychological dysfunction in the workplace: normative data from the Pittsburgh occupational exposures test battery. J *Clin Exp Neuropsychol*. 1987;9:666-679.

7. Morrow LA, et al. Psychiatric symtomatology in persons with organic solvent exposure. J *Consult Clin Psychol*. 1993;51:171-4

8. Morrow LA, et al. Risk factors associated with persistence of neuropsychological deficits in persons with organic solvent exposure. J *Nervous Mental Disease*. 1991;179(9):540-545.

9. Morrow LA. Assessment of attention and memory

efficiency in persons with solvent neurotoxicity. *Neuropsychologia.* 1992;30(10):911-922.

10. Morrow LA, et al. A distinct pattern of personality disturbance following exposure to mixtures of organic solvents. *J Occup Med.* 1989;31(9):743-745.

11. *Pesticides in Diets of Infants and Children.* Washington, DC:National Research Council, National Academy Press;1993:3.

12. *Neurotoxicity: Identifying and Controlling Poisons of the Nervous System.* Washington, DC: Superintendent of Documents, Government Printing Office; April 1990:44. GPO Stock #052-003-01184-1.

13. Weiss B. Environmental contaminants and behavioral disorders. *J Develop Pharm Ther.* 1967;10:346-353.

14. Chester AC, Levine PH. Concurrent Sick Building Syndrome and Chronic Fatigue Syndrome: Epidemic Neuromyasthenia Revised. *Clinical Infectious Diseases.* 1994;18:S43-S48

15. *Environmental Hazards in Your School, A Resource Handbook.* Washington, DC:US Environmental Protection Agency; October 1990. Publication #201-2001.

16. Wilkenfeld IR. Contaminated classrooms: when learning becomes lethal. *Townsend Letter for Doctors.* 1993;1:114-118.

17 Wilkenfeld IR. School construction should include attention to air quality. *South Bend Tribune* (Indiana). August 9.1994: A-9

18. Savage EP, et al. Chronic neurological sequelae of acute organophosphate pesticide poisoning. *Arch Environ Health.* 1988;43(1):38-45.

19. Korsek RJ, Sato MM. Effects of chronic organophosphate pesticide exposure on the central nervous system. Clin Toxicol. 1977;11(1):83-95.

20. Rodnitzky RL. Behavioral effects of organophosphate pesticides in man. Clin Toxicol. 1976;9(3):391-405.

21. Dési I. Neurotoxicological investigation of pesticides in animal experiments. Neurobehav Toxicol Teratol. 1983;5:503-515.

22. Gershon S, Shaw FH. Psychiatric sequelae of chronic exposure to organophosphorus insecticides. Lancet. June 24, 1981:1371-1374.

23. Tabershaw IR, Cooper WC. Sequelae of acute organic phosphate poisoning. J Occup Med. 1988;8(1):8-20.

24. Durham WF, et al. Organophosphorus insecticides and mental alertness. Arch Environ Health. 1985;10:55-68.

25. Dille JR, Smith PW. Central nervous system effects of chronic exposure to organophosphate insecticides. Aerospace Med. May 1984:476-478

26. Rodnitzky RL, Lavin SH, Mick DL. Occupational exposure to organophosphate pesticides. Arch Environ Health. 1975;30:98-103.

27. Rodnitzky RL, Lavin SH, Mick DL. Anxiety associated with exposure to organophosphate compounds. Arch Gen Psychiatry. 1976;33:225-228.

28. Hardman PK, Lieberman A, Preston P. *Academic behavioral, and perceptual reactions in dyslexic children when exposed to environmental factors: malathion and petrochemical ethanol.* Tallahassee, FL: Dyslexia Research Institute; 1981.

29. *Intolerable Risk: Pesticides in Our Children's Foods.* Washington, DC:Natural Resources Defense Council; February 27, 1989:71-98.

31. Ecobichon D, Joy RM: *Pesticides and Neurologic Diseases.* Boca Raton, FL:CRC Press;1982:171.

32. Desi I. Neurotoxicological investigation of pesticides in animal experiments. *Neurobehav Tox Teratol.* 1983;8:

33. Hodgson AT, et al. Emissions of volatile organic compounds from new carpets measured in a large-scale environmental laboratory. J *Air Waste Management Assoc.* 1993;43(3):316-324.

34 Melnick RL, Huff J. 1,3-Butadiene: toxicity and carcinogenicity in laboratory animals and humans. *Rev Environmental Contam Toxic.* 1992;124:111-144.

35. Landrigan P. Critical assessment of epidemiologic studies on the human carcinogenicity of 1,3-Butadiene. *Envir Health Perspect.* 1990;86:143-147.

36. Swanson J. *The Psychological and Educational Implications of Formaldehyde Toxicology.* Thesis. University of Northern Colorado;1984

37. Bear D, et al. Aggression in cat and human precipitated by an acetylcholine esterase inhibitor. *Psychomatics.* 1988;27(7):535-538.

Valuable sources of information

Berthold-Bond A. *Clean & Green.* Woodstock, NY:Ceres Press; 1990.

Bower J. *The Healthy House - How to Buy One.-.How to Cure a "Sick" One.-.How to Build One.* Secaucus, NJ:Lyle Stuart;1989
Common-Sense Pest Control. Available from the Bio-Integral Resource Center, P.O. Box 7414, Berkeley, CA 94707, (510) 524-2567, 1991.

Dadd DL. *The Nontoxic Home & Office.* New York:G.P. Putman's Sons; 1992.

Dadd DL. *Nontoxic, Natural, and Earthwise.* Los Angeles: Jeremy P. Thatcher; 1990.

Dadd DL. *The Nontoxic Home.* Los Angeles:Thatcher Inc., distributed by St. Martin's Press, New York, 1986.

Dadd DL. *Nontoxic & Natural.* Los Angeles:Thatcher; 1984.

Environmental Hazards in Your School: A Resource Handbook. Washington, DC:United States Environmental Protection Agency; 1990. Publication #201-2001.

Gorman CP. *Less-Toxic Living. Environmental Health Center:* 8345 Walnut Hill Lane, Suite 205, Dallas, Texas 75231, (214) 368-4132.

Health House Catalog. Cleveland, OH:Environmental Health Watch and the Housing Resource Center; 1990.

The Inside Story.-.A Guide to Indoor Air Quality. Washington, DC:United States Environmental Protection Agency; 1988: EPA/400/1-88/004.

Lawson L. *Staying Well in a Toxic World.* Chicago; Noble Press:1993:(Note: If we were limited to a single choice encompassing the field of environmental hazards with guidelines for their avoidance, this book would be our choice.)

Miller NL, ed. *The Healthy School Handbook.* Washington, DC:National Education Association; 1995:
(*Order from:* NEA Professional Library, PO Box 509, West Haven, CT 06516, $15.95.)

Rousseau D, Rea W. *Your Home, Your Health, and Well-Being.* Cleveland, OH:Environmental Health Watch; 1989:
The Healthy House Institute Headed by John Bower, author of The

Healthy House listed above and an expert in safe building materials and procedures, offers valuable monographs and consultations in building problems. The address is 7471 N. Shiloh Rd., Unionville, IN 47468, (812)-332-5073.

CHAPTER 6
The importance of light for the hyperactive child

One of the more neglected areas in care of the child involves lack of exposure to natural sunlight and poor quality indoor lighting The latter often consists of cool-white fluorescent lights in schools and day care centers. The cool-white fluorescent tubes put out a limited color spectrum in contrast to full spectrum fluorescent tubes or, of course, natural sunlight.

The importance of full spectrum lighting was demonstrated in 1973 by John Ott, a leading pioneer in the field of lighting. He conducted an experiment in which he compared the effects of full spectrum lighting with cool-white fluorescent lighting on students in separate classrooms in Sarasota, Florida. Concealed, time-lapse cameras recorded sequences of student activity. The results were significant. In cool-white fluorescent light, some students demonstrated hyperactivity, fatigue, irritability, and attention deficits. In contrast, in another class , behavior, and as well as overall academic achievement, showed marked improvement within one month after full spectrum lighting was installed . Furthermore, several learning-disabled students with extreme hyperactivity problems miraculously calmed down, and seemed to overcome some of their learning and reading problems, while in the classrooms with full spectrum lighting.[1]

We tend to think of air, food, and water as the three essentials for life. We forget there could be no life on earth without sunlight. Although our knowledge in this area is in a very early stage, indirect sun rays come through the eyes and affect the pineal gland and its production of melatonin. This in turn affects or governs the hypothalamus and through the hypothalamus the endocrine systems of the body.[2]

As a basic guideline, it is desirable for everyone to spend at least one hour per day out-of-doors, but it is especially important for children to do so.

References

1. Lieberman J. Light, Medicine of the Future. Santa Fe, NM: Bear & Co.1991:58

2. Lieberman J. Light, Medicine of the Future. Santa Fe, Santa Fe, NM: Bear & Co. 1991:Chap 2,10

CHAPTER 7
Water pollution

It was largely in the 1970s and early 1980s that the extensive industrial pollution of water supplies was disclosed and that corrective efforts began to take place. Examples included the heavy contamination of Great Lakes areas with mercury and deadly polychlorinated biphenyls (PCB's), dioxins in Love Canal at Niagara Falls, and leakage from underground gasoline storage tanks.[1]

In spite of attempted corrective measures, chemical water pollution remains a widespread problem. Traces of numerous volatile organic chlorinated compounds are commonly present.[2] Nitrates, which can be dangerous for babies, have been found to be the number one contaminant in Pennsylvania, originating from fertilizers in farming areas.[3]

Plumbing systems may also be the source of chemicals in drinking water. Recently, lead in solder has been limited to trace amounts and is not considered a problem in new installations, but in older systems, solder may be a source of lead. Plastic pipe is now used more frequently because of lower cost. These polybutylene or polyvinyl chloride pipes may give off toxic gases. The solvents and glues used with plastic lines may also be problematic.[4]

Water testing

Commercial testing of drinking water can also be done in many laboratories, but it is important to know just which chemicals to select for testing, as the pollutants could number in the hundreds, making comprehensive testing extremely expensive.

Local or State Health Boards often provide some testing at no charge, or reasonable cost, if there is medical evidence of health risk. Usually, they will do health screening for the most likely pollutants such as formaldehyde, petrochemicals, lead, and organic compounds. If additional tests are needed, the telephone directory under Laboratories or Board of Health may provide a list of commercial laboratories.

Alternative solutions

The first solution, one which many families undertake, is to purchase high quality spring water in glass bottles for drinking or cooking. The purity of the water should be checked, for not all commercial suppliers of bottled water are from genuine, unpolluted spring sources.

Second, commercial water filters are now available

at reasonable cost. These can be attached to the kitchen faucet for water used for drinking and cooking.

Third, water can be brought to a boil and then allowed to stand and cool overnight in an open pan or jar. This will drive out the volatile chemicals but will not eliminate metals such as lead or the fluoride from water fluoridation.

References

1. Beasely J, Swift JJ. *The Kellogg Report*. Annondale-On-Hudson, NY: The Institute of Health Policy and Practice, Bard College Center. 1989:185-186.

2. Wallace LA, et al. The TEAM study: personal exposures to toxic substances in air, drinking water, and breath of 400 residents of New Jersey, North Carolina, and North Dakota. *Environm. Research*. 1987;43: 290-307.

3. Dore C. Water on tap gets a bad rap. *The Daily Intelligencer.*(Doylestown, PA) February 23, 1996.

4. Bower J. *The Healthy House*. New York, NY: Lyle Stuart. 1989:307-309.

CHAPTER 8
Toxic heavy metals: lead, cadmium, mercury, antimony and aluminum.

Although other metals can be toxic under certain circumstances, lead, cadmium, mercury, antimony and aluminum are generally considered to be foremost in public health concerns. There is far more awareness of the health hazards from these toxic metals than from the volatile organic compounds, and therefore there is considerable progress in toxic metals control. Nevertheless, they still remain a health threat to the public, especially to children.

Lead

Numerous reports have shown that lead exposures in children can result in Intelligence quotient (IQ) deficits.[1,2] The incidence of documented lead toxicity in children has declined substantially since leaded gasoline was phased out in the early 1980s. Six potential sources for lead exposure remain:

- Flaking lead paint in older buildings: Houses or apartments built before 1950 are almost certain to have lead paint on their walls. When construction occurred between 1950 and 1980, chances are about 50-50 that lead is present (although lead paint from houses was banned after 1972). Do-it-yourself lead testing kits are available for between $35.00 and $50.00.
- Tap water in older buildings with lead pipes or in newer buildings in which lead solder was used to seal connections in the plumbing.
- Outdoor soil contamination as a fallout from earlier years when leaded gasoline was used. Incompletely washed fruits and vegetables may contain traces of this contaminated soil. Another major source is outdoor dust blowing into houses.
- Activities involving lead solder.
- Some art supplies. Although lead has been outlawed for most paints, it is not outlawed in artist's paints.
- Prolonged exposure at pistol and rifle firing ranges.

Older houses should be checked for lead. If lead paint is present, alternatives include removal of the paint, which should always be done by professionals with protective gear, or to repaint the surfaces, sealing in the older paint (check with local building codes).

It is probably advisable to check tap water for

lead, unless it is certain there is no lead in the plumbing. Fruits and vegetables should be washed thoroughly. Houses should be kept free of dust.

Cadmium

Cadmium, a neurotoxin, has been implicated in mental retardation.[3] Increased levels have been found in placentas of mothers who smoke and may cause low birthweight in babies.[4] Children and pregnant women should not be exposed to passive tobacco smoking from second-hand smoke. Cadmium may also come from tap water when cadmium alloys have been used for soldering plumbing joints.

Mercury

Mercury is a neurotoxin. It tends to accumulate in the body and is not easily expelled. The classical neurologic and disordered behavioral symptoms of mercury poisoning are exhibited in *Alice in Wonderland* by the Mad Hatter. For hatters in the Victorian era, mercury poisoning was an occupational hazard.

In 1989, the EPA banned mercury from indoor paints after the case of a four year old boy made severely ill as a result of indoor paint exposure. However, exterior coatings are still allowed to contain mercury, and stored paint manufactured before the ban may also contain mercury. (National Pesticide Telecommunication Network at 800-858-7378 maintains a listing of older paints that may contain mercury.)

Perhaps the most controversial and lively issue concerning mercury today surrounds the silver/mercury dental fillings. According to reports, mercury constitutes about 50% of these fillings. Because mercury vaporizes above 10°F, an estimated 3 to 17 mcg of mercury are absorbed daily into the system from mercury amalgams. The new composite, porcelain, or ceramic fillings should be used for all future dental work.

Antimony

High levels of antimony, sometimes used as a flame-retardant in pillows and mattresses, has been found in children with autism with significant frequency, according to Jon Pangborn, PhD, in his research report delivered at the Autism Research Institute Conference in Chicago in June of 1996.

Aluminum

Aluminum is a relative newcomer to the list of toxic metals, long having been considered harmless. It has been implicated as a contributory cause of Alzheimer's disease.[5] Elevated hair aluminum in children, especially when attended with elevations of lead, have been found to cause decreased visual-motor performance.[6]

We routinely recommend hair tests for ADHD children, primarily as a screening test for lead. Rather surprisingly, the most consistent finding is that of elevated hair aluminum.

Aluminum comes from foods cooked or stored in aluminum pans and aluminum foil. Leafy vegetables, rhubarb, and apples cooked in aluminum pans are prone to leach the metal from the pan. Pressure cookers are especially likely to impart metal into the food. Tap water may contain aluminum when it is used in water reservoirs to flocculate silt from the water. Other sources include antacids taken for stomach trouble, some antiperspirants, food additives, and milk substitutes.

Clinical management of toxic heavy metals

We employ the hair test in screening for heavy metals, although blood tests for lead should also be done in ADHD and learning disabled children. When elevated levels are found, the first responsibility is to seek and eliminate the source as much as possible. When blood lead exceeds 10 mcg, the child should be referred to a medical center for appropriate therapy. This, however, is increasingly uncommon - we have yet to see a single case with this level.

Except in the more severe cases of heavy metal toxicity, we believe treatment should be nutritional, which works slowly but effectively and safely. Even here, if a child is ill and heavy metals are suspected as a contributory cause, treatment should not be attempted without professional guidance.

Treatment measures may include, but are not limited to, the following:

- Vitamin C: increases the turnover rate of toxic metals and reduces damage by scavenging free radicals generated by the toxins.[7]
- Sulfur-containing amino acids from sulfur-rich food such as garlic, onions, beans, and lentils.act as chelating or binding agents for the heavy metals,forming relatively inert bonds with the heavy metals, in which form they can be carried out of the body.[8]
- Vitamin B1 (thiamin) contains a sulfide-containing thiazole ring, which acts in a similar manner.
- Sulfide-containing amino acids: glutathione may be the most valuable.
- In addition to garlic seasoning in foods, garlic capsules can be given.
- Nutrient trace minerals including calcium,magnesium, zinc, manganese, copper, selenium, and iron, given as supplements, are of utmost importance in treating the child with heavy metal toxicity for two reasons. First, such a child will almost invariably be deficient in these minerals and, second, these minerals (especially calcium, zinc, copper, and iron) tend literally - to push the toxic metals out of the body as they are replenished.[8]
- Blue-green algae or chlorella, taken as oral supplements, may be the single most effective preventive measure against mercury toxicity. Taken in combinationtion with garlic, these supplements provide a

rich supply of sulfhydryl groups, which combine with mercury and help to move it from its intracellular storage positions while at the same time disarming its toxicity. Research, although still in its early phases, tends to confirm this role.

It may not be inappropriate to end this chapter with a true story told by an attorney, Jon Pangborn at the Autism Research Institute Conference in June of 1996: Some years ago, there was a company in which employees had been made ill by lead exposure. The employees sued the company. The company's defense rested on one man, more directly exposed than other employees, who remained perfectly healthy. The company's attorney argued that if this man were not ill, then lead could not be the cause of illness in the others. As it turned out, the man in question was a Mexican. What do Mexicans eat? They eat beans. In this case, they protected the Mexican from the lead. When this knowledge was revealed, presumably the other employees won their case.

References

1. Air Quality Criteria for Lead. Research Triangle Park. NC: US Environmental Protection Agency; 1986. 4 volumes. EPA-600/8-83 028aF.

2. Needleman HL, et al. Deficits in psychological and classroom performance of children with elevated dentine lead levels. N Engl J Med. 1979;300:689-693.

3. Marlow M, et al. Hair mineral content as a predictor of mental retardation. OrthoPsych. 1983;12(1):26-33.

4. Miller J, et al.;Haley, Berndt, ed Reproductive & perinatal toxicology. Handbook of Toxicology. Washington, DC.

5. Martyn CN, et al. Geographical relation between Alzheimer's disease and aluminum in drinking water. Lancet. 1989;1:59-62.

6. Moon C, et al. Main and interaction effects of metallic pollutants on cognitive functioning. J Learning Disabilities. 1985;18:217-221..

7. Hume AS, et al. Binding of toxicants by carbonyl & sulfide containing chemicals. Environ Med. 1991;8(3):96-100.

8. Isaacson RL, Jensen KF, eds. The Vulnerable Brain and Environmental Risks. Vol 2. New York:Plenum Press; 1992:118-120.

Recommended reading:

Casdorph HR, Walker M. Toxic Metal Syndrome: How Metal Poisonings Can Affect Your Brain. Stamford, CT: Freelance Communications;1994.

CHAPTER 9
Fluoridation: pros and cons

Fluoride may now be added to the list of potentially neurotoxic chemicals as indicated by a recent study conducted at Harvard Medical School, Eastman Dental Center, Iowa State University and Forsythe Research Institute. According to this study, the first of its kind, fluoride carries the potential for "motor dysfunction, IQ deficits and/or learning disabilities in humans.[1]"

Fluoride began to be added to municipal water supplies that were low in fluoride in the 1940s after a study sponsored by the US Public Health Service indicated that adding one part per million of fluoride reduced tooth decay. Today, approximately half of the population in the United States drinks water from municipal supplies that have been artificially fluoridated.[2] Additional sources of fluoride include fluoride-containing toothpastes, vitamin and mineral supplements with fluoride for children, and dental applications.

There has been a decline in tooth decay in recent decades, but the role of fluoride in this decline remains controversial. The American Dental Association, which has steadfastly promoted fluoridation, credits fluoridation with the decline. However, in the text, *Fluoride, The Aging Factor*, Dr. John Yiamouyiannis, extensively reviewed the subject. He pointed out extensive studies showing that fluoridation of water supplies has been ineffective in preventing dental decay with equal incidence in fluoridated and nonfluoridated communities.[3,4] As reported by Yiamouyiannis, scientists at the US Environmental Protection Agency have come out against water fluoridation because they have confirmed that fluoridation does not reduce tooth decay and that there is clear evidence that fluoridation causes cancer.[5] Animal studies showing fluoride-linked increases in bone cancer and oral cancer have been confirmed by human studies.[6] He also points out that the US Centers for Disease Control and the British Health Ministry admit that no laboratory study has shown that the amount of fluoride added to drinking water is effective in reducing tooth decay.[7]

The only form of fluoride that may be effective in reducing dental decay, according to Yiamouyiannis, is that found in toothpaste.[8] Fluoride's principal decay preventive action is on the surface of the teeth.[9] The downside of fluoridated toothpaste is that, according to a study at the Madras Dental

College, India, even small amounts of fluoridated toothpaste are quickly absorbed into the general circulation.[10]

Even if topical applications of fluoride to teeth do reduce dental caries, what adverse health effects are there from fluoride accumulations in the body as a result of multiple exposures as is commonly the case, especially for children? The Yiamouyiannis text, always well documented, points out the following complications:

- **Cancer:** Epidemiological surveys consistently have shown increased incidence of cancer in fluoridated cities as compared with nonfluoridated cities.[11]

- **Defective bone formation:** Although fluoride-stimulated bone is denser, it is structurally unsound and more prone to fractures. A variety of medical studies have reported increased hip fractures in the elderly in communities with fluoridated water.[12-15]

- **Premature aging of skin, arteries, and other tissues:** By damaging or disrupting connective tissue and collagen, fluoride tends to promote calcification (hardening) of arteries and ligaments and wrinkling of skin.[16]

- **Disarming the immune system:** Researchers studying fluoride tissue levels in patients living in fluoridated areas, have found distortions in the body's proteins resulting in autoimmune or allergic responses. There was also reduced migration of white blood cells (the body's immune defense system) and reduced ability of white blood cells to attack invading organisms.[17]

- **Genetic damage:** It is clear that fluoride is capable of causing genetic damage, according to Yiamouyiannis, although the exact mechanism cannot be pinpointed because fluoride interferes with a number of physiologic processes.[18]

- **Impaired memory:** The ability of fluoride to interfere with enzyme activity at 1 ppm or less is not a point of controversy. The US National Academy of Sciences, the World Health Organization (WHO) and others have published lists of enzymes that are inhibited at 1 ppm or less. One of these is the enzyme acetylcholinesterase.[19] This enzyme produces the neurotransmitter, acetyl choline, which transmits nerve impulses in the brain and peripheral nervous system and therefore is involved in learning and memory. Because fluoride inhibits the enzyme, acetylcholinesterase, there would be less thought and less memory. The situation is analogous to an electrical circuit. The bigger the wire (more acetyl choline), the less the electrical resistance. The smaller the wire (less acetylcholine due to fluoride), then more electrical resistance (slower thought).

In conclusion, one of the surveys showing no benefit from water fluoridation in tooth decay came from New Zealand.[20] The authors commented that a decline in tooth decay had commenced before the introduction of any form of fluoride. The decline was attributed to changes in diet, such as increased consumption of fresh fruits, vegetables, and cheese, which is known to be tooth decay inhibiting. One might surmise there was also a reduction in sugar with its well-recognized decay-causing propensities.

In our opinion, the adverse effects of fluoridation far outweigh the meager benefits of its purported reduction in tooth decay. Instead, we should rely primarily on a healthy diet.

References

1. Mullenix PJ, et al. Neurotoxicity of sodium fluoride in rats. Neurotox & Teratol. 1995;17:169-177.

2. Disendorf M. Have the benefits of water fluoridation been overestimated? Int Clin Nutr Rev. 1990;10(2):292-303.

3. Yiamouyiannis J. Fluoride,The Aging Factor. Delaware, OH:Health Action Press; 1993:Chap 14.

4. Diesendorf M. The mystery of declining tooth decay. Nature. 1986;322:125-129.

5. Yiamouyiannis J. Fluoride,The Aging Factor.. Delaware, OH:Health Action Press; 1993:204-208.

6. Yiamouyiannis J. Fluoride,The Aging Factor. Delaware, OH:Health Action Press; 1993:123.

7. Yiamouyiannis J. Fluoride,The Aging Factor. Delaware, OH:Health Action Press; 1993:132.

8. Werbach MR. Nutritional influences in illness - fluoride. Townsend Letter for Doctors. Aug/Sept 1994:853.

9. Douglas WC. Second Opinion. 1994;IV(4):1.

10. Yiamouyiannis J. Fluoride,Fluoride, The Aging Factor. Delaware, OH:Health Action Press; 1993:85-87.

11. Yiamouyiannis J. Fluoride,The Aging Factor. Delaware, OH:Health Action Press; 1993:Chap 9.

12. Lindsay R. Fluoride and bone - quantity versus quality. N Engl J Med. Editorial. 1990;322(12):845-846.

13. Colquhoun J. Fluoridation: new evidence of harm to young teeth and bones. Int Clin Nutr Rev. 1992;12(10):1-8.

14. Jacobsen S, et al. Regional variation in the incidence of hip fracture. JAMA. 1990;264:500-502.

15. Riggs BL. Effect of fluoride treatment on the fracture rate in postmenopausal women with osteoporosis. N Engl J Med. 1990;322:802-809.

16. Yiamouyiannis J. Fluoride, The Aging Factor.. Delaware, OH:Health Action Press; 1993:Chap 7.

17. Yiamouyiannis J. Fluoride, The Aging Factor. Delaware, OH:Health Action Press; 1993:Chap 3.

18. Yiamouyiannis J. Fluoride, The Aging Factor. Delaware, OH:Health Action Press; 1993:Chap 8.

19. Yiamouyiannis J. Fluoride, the Aging Factor. Delaware, OH:Health Action Press; 1993:91-92.

20. Colquhoun J. FluoridesOur toxic world - Who is looking after our kids? and the decline in tooth decay in New Zealand. Fluoride. 1993;26(2):125-134.1.

CHAPTER 10
Overuse of antibiotics and the need for alternatives

In future times, medical historians may write the following epitaph about the field of antibiotic therapy: "died of overuse."

Articles in popular news magazines based on interviews with authorities at leading medical centers quote estimates that over half of antibiotic use in the United States is unnecessary and inappropriate.[1,2]

There are good reasons for concern about the present level of antibiotic usage.

1. **Suppression of the immune system by antibiotics:**

Even a cursory search of medical literature concerning the immune-suppressant effects of antibiotics will reveal a flow of published scientific studies in the past several decades showing depression of various arms of the immune system by antibiotics. One clinical report illustrating this effect involved a study of 460 children with middle-ear infections with fluid build-up (secretory otitis media) in which a portion of the children were treated with the antibiotic, Amoxicillin,® and a portion were treated with an inactive placebo. According to the authors, children treated with Amoxicillin® *were two to six times more likely to have another ear infection within the next six weeks*, presumably the result of immunosuppression caused by the antibiotic.[3] Furthermore, children treated with the placebo were equally likely to be well four weeks later. Because of this and similar studies, 1994 guidelines for treating children with secretory otitis media call for a period of observation of three or four months rather than immediate antibiotic therapy.[4]

2. Overgrowth of potentially harmful bacteria, yeast and mold:

The healthy intestinal tract might aptly be compared with a garden. Beneficial microorganisms (bacteria) predominate, many of which are essential to life and health. Potentially harmful (pathogenic) microorganisms such as *Staphylococcus*, *Clostridium*, and yeast forms could be compared with weeds of a garden. These are kept in check as long as the beneficial bacteria flourish. However, when antibiotics are given, there may be a major shift in balance with a killing out of large numbers of the beneficial bacteria. This, in turn, potentially allows overgrowth of the pathogens. Although the adverse effects may not be immediately apparent, there may be a long-term deterioration of health with increased illness and allergies.[5-10]

In addition, it should be noted that the healthful bacteria produce lactic acid, which tends to inhibit growth of harmful yeast and fungi. When the source of lactic acid is reduced by killing off of the beneficial bacteria by antibiotics, the yeast and mold may proliferate. This can result in various forms of ill health.

3. Promotion of antibiotic-resistant microorganisms:

There is a steadily growing incidence of antibiotic-resistant infectious diseases, promoted not only by medical usage of antibiotics but also by their use in the food industry.[1,2] Infections such as pneumonia, septicemia (blood poisoning), gonorrhea, syphilis, tuberculosis, and *Staphylococcus* are becoming increasing difficult to treat and, sometimes, are not in reach of the strongest medications. If the process continues several more decades, it is possible that many common infections of today will be beyond reach of even the strongest antibiotics.

A practical plan:

Antibiotics should be avoided in uncomplicated viral infections such as colds and influenza (viruses are immune to the effects of antibiotics). The same should hold for uncomplicated secretory otitis media in children. If time and effort are taken to use some of the "natural" approaches outlined below. Complications can be avoided in a majority of instances. However, if potentially serious complications do ensue and antibiotics become necessary, then there should be no stint in the dosage. Take the full course recommended by your doctor; anything else will favor the emergence of drug-resistant germs. When in doubt concerning the seriousness of an infection, consult your physician.

Two measures will help to counteract the adverse effects of antibiotics, should these become necessary:

1. Take some commercial preparation with *Lactobacillus acidophilus* and *bifidis*, healthful bacteria normally present in the digestive tract, to replace those killed by the antibiotic. It may be started before completion of the course of antibiotics and continued possibly several weeks afterwards.

2. Take a serving of plain, unflavored yogurt daily. Yogurt contains lactic acid, which will help to keep the pathogens in check. (An exception for the use of yogurt is noted below).

Eat lightly
Heavy foods, especially rich desserts, tend to burden the immune system, contribute to inflammation, and create mucus. If there is a buildup of mucus in the sinuses, middle ear, or chest, avoid milk products, including yogurt. Milk tends to promote mucus production in the body.11. According to folk tradition, chicken soup may contain biological ingredients that

reduce the body's inflammation response. Adding garlic, which also has anti-inflammatory properties, may add to this response.

"Natural" remedies should be used at the earliest sign of a cold or influenza. Although many natural approaches to healing have prompted a surprising amount of credible scientific research, it is true that they are seldom favored by the same level of scientific research required for pharmaceuticals by US laws. For this reason, natural healing and folk medicine are commonly referred to as unscientific. This depends on the point of view. There is another frame of reference, that of common experience and observation. A good rule is that if an approach in folk medicine has survived two or more generations in two or more societies, it has survived the test of time, which may be as high a level of scientific evaluation as the favored double-blind study of today.

Finally, get plenty of rest when ill. Few things will lower the resistance quicker than inadequate rest and sleep.

Natural remedies from the lore of folk medicine for colds and influenza

- As suggested by Julian Whitaker, MD, slice one or two cloves of garlic and blend them with 8 oz of orange or grapefruit juice with a bit of lemon. Drink two glasses between meals, or one glass as a substitute for a meal. Clinical studies have shown that garlic possesses both antibacterial and antiviral properties.

- Drink several glasses of spring water daily in addition to the fruit juice.
- Take about 1,000 mg vitamin C per waking hour. Cut back if it causes diarrhea. Reduce doses in children proportionate to weight, such as half dose for a 75-pound child, quarter dose for a 40-pound child, and so on.
- Take zinc lozenges about four times daily for about a week. Zinc enhances the immune system and has antiviral activity. Do not take longer than a week because dosage over longer periods may suppress the immune system.
- Take medicinal herbs such as echinacea, myrrh, and/or goldenseal, all of which enhance the immune system. Doses should be one dropper full of the tincture or one capsule of powdered form four times daily, continued 7 to 10 days. If continued for prolonged periods, they lose their effectiveness. Reduce children's doses in proportion to their weights.

For upset stomach: Ginger and/or camomile tea.

For persistent cough: Elecampane tea.

For diarrhea: Goldenseal as tea, tincture, or capsule.

For fluid buildup in the middle ear with mild inflammation: Ear drops containing mullein oil and garlic.

For eye inflammation: Eyebright tea.

For sore throats: Gargle with hydrogen peroxide (available from drug stores) mixed half and half with water.

Once again, it should be emphasized that these remedies are recommended for minor viral infections in the absence of potentially serious bacterial complications. For children, parents are urged to use equal portions of observation, common sense, and intuition to judge when medical intervention is required and they need to call the doctor. However, if these simple though possibly time-consuming measures are followed, experience has shown that the incidence of complications from viral infections will be greatly reduced, thereby reducing the need for antibiotics.

Future trends:

As a straw-in-the-wind for future trends, a nine-month survey begun in 1994 of nearly 700 children, showed a disturbing link between developmental delays in children and antibiotics usage.[12]

The survey, was conducted by the Developmental Delay Registry, of their multi-national database of 800 families, most of which have children with developmental delays. It found.that children who had taken more than 20 cycles of antibiotics in their lifetime were over 50% more likely to suffer developmental delays than children taking fewer than three cycles of antibiotics.

The survey's other findings include:

- Nearly 75% of the delayed children were reported to be developing normally in their first year of life.
- Children who took 20 cycles of antibiotics were twice as likely to have ear tube infections than children taking fewer than three cycles of antibiotics.
- Children who took 20 cycles of antibiotics were nearly four times more likely to have had negative reactions to immunizations.

These findings are, at best, preliminary and should be interpreted with caution. Their importance is that they may be among the early indications of a historic change in direction in health and medical research.

References

1. Freedman DH. Good drugs, dangerous doses. *Reader's Digest.* May 1994:142-144.

2. Begley S. The end of antibiotics. *Newsweek.* March 28, 1994:47-52.

3. Cantekin EI, et al. *JAMA.* 1991;266:3309.

4. Kritz F. Otitis approach conservative. *Medical Tribune.* Aug 11, 1994:1.

5. Melby K, Midvedt T. Effects of some antibacterial agents on phagocytosis of 33-P-labeled *Escherichia coli* by human polymorphonuclear cells. *Acta Pathol Microbiol.* Scandinavian Section B.88:1980;103-106.

6. Seelig MJ. Role of antibiotic in the pathogenesis of *Candida* infections. *Am J Med.* 1996;40:887-917.

7. Seelig MJ. The rationale for preventing antibacterial-induced fungal overgrowth. *Medical Times.* 1968;9(7): 689-710.

8. Trowbridge JP. *The Yeast Syndrome.* New York, NY: Bantam Books; 1986:42-54.

9. Voiculescu C, et al. Experimental study of antibiotic-induced immunosuppression in mice. *Comp Immun Microbiol Infect Dis.* 1983;6(4):291-299.

10. Seelig MJ. Mechanisms by which antibiotics increase the incidence and severity of candidiasis and alter the immunological defenses. *Bacteriol Rev.* 1968;30(2).

11. Collins AM, et al. Bovine milk, including pasteurized milk, contains antibodies directed against allergens of clinical importance to man. *Int Arch Allergy Appl Immuno.* 1991;96:362-367.

12. Developmental Delay Registry (DDR) *is located at* PO Box 12394, Silver Spring MD 20908. (301) 924-3060. Fax: (301) 654-0557

Recommended reading

Iappe M. *When Antibiotics Fail: Restoring the Ecology of the Body.* Berkeley, CA: North Atlantic Books; 1986.

Schmidt MA. *Childhood Ear Infections: What Every Parent and Physician Should Know about Prevention, Home Care, and Alternate Treatment.* Berkeley, CA: North Atlantic Books.1990

Schmidt MA, Smith LH, Sehnert KW. *Beyond Antibiotics: Healthier Options for Families.* Berkeley, CA: North Atlantic Books; 1993.

Chapter 11
Current childhood vaccination programs: do they cause more disease than they prevent?

It is unpleasant but necessary to point out that there are now serious trends of increasing health problems among American children. Allergic diseases such as eczema and asthma are increasing both in frequency and severity. As one example, surveys have shown a 46% increase nationwide in deaths from asthma between 1977 and 1991.[1] Asthma among children has increased 200% in the past 20 years.[2] Ear, sinus, throat, and bronchial infections are occurring on a scale unknown in earlier generations. Young parents have commented to me that, a majority of the children of their friends and acquaintances,are on antibiotics frequently or, in some instances, continually. It was not like this even 20 or 30 years ago. With each passing year, there appear to be manifestations of increasing crippling of children's immune systems. Surveys among elementary school teachers confirm this trends.[3]

Among young adults the chronic fatigue syndrome, now recognized to be an immunologic disorder[4] is widespread. Autoimmune diseases, those in which the immune system attacks the body's own cells and tissues, are also increasing.

No one knows the full answer for these unfortunate trends, but there is now a great deal of evidence that current childhood vaccine programs may be one of the underlying causes.[5,6]

The time is long overdue to rethink the entire matter of ongoing mass childhood vaccinations. It is a general impression that the vaccines played a major role in controlling infectious diseases which, in earlier times, decimated populations of children. This is doubtful. As carefully reviewed in the text on vaccinations by Viera Scheibner, PhD,[6] these diseases had declined by up to 90% before any vaccine was used in mass proportions. Dr. Scheibner further cast doubt on the effectiveness of the vaccines by reporting recent epidemics of measles and whooping cough in fully vaccinated children. In view of the valid questions about the efficacy of modern vaccines and growing concerns about harmful side effects, which appear to be greatly underestimated, an objective reappraisal is needed.

Basic concerns about current childhood vaccines:

1. Multiple vaccines during early infancy:

Current vaccine programs call for numerous vaccines during the first six months of life. It would appear it is taken for granted that the immune reservoir of the infant has an unlimited capacity to respond to these vaccines, but this is far from the case. The newborn comes into the world with a highly immature and undeveloped immune system which does not ordinarily become fully developed until about 12 years of age. The process of maturation requires a series of natural infectious challenges to become mature and strong. According to standard pediatric texts these are spaced an average of once every six weeks, the great majority of which occur without illness.

The host of simultaneous vaccines given repeatedly over a short period of time comprise a wide variant from this natural spacing of challenges. Also, all vaccines, with the exception of one which is given orally, are injected directly by needles into the system, thereby bypassing the mucosal immune system (the Secretory IgA system) of the respiratory and gastrointestinal systems which otherwise would cushion a large majority of infectious challenges. It is difficult to conceive that these intensive challenges would not over stimulate and use up the highly immature and undeveloped immune capacity of the infant to an abnormal extent, leaving it more vulnerable to other infections. As observed by Coulter Harris, it may be more than coincidental that a host of infections often follow these vaccines.[7]

Viral vaccines have been shown to depress cellular immunity,[8,9] which serves as the body's first line of defense against infections. In 1984 a little noted letter was published in *the New England Journal of Medicine*[10] which reported a significant, though temporary drop of T-helper lymphocytes in 11 healthy adults given routine tetanus vaccinations. In explanation, the T-helper lymphocytes are a class of white blood cells which help to govern the immune system. Special concern rests in the fact that drops in T-helper lymphocytes are characteristic of acquired immune deficiency syndrome (AIDS), and in four of the 11 recipients of the tetanus vaccine the T-helper lymphocytes dropped to levels seen in active AIDS patients.

This was the effect in healthy adults. One must wonder what the effects of multiple vaccines given to infants must be on various parameters of the immune system, but as far as I am aware, this has not been tested.

2. Live virus vaccines incubated in animal tissues

Live virus vaccines require incubation in animal tissues. The oral polio vaccine is incubated in monkey kidneys and the MMR (measles, mumps, rubella) vaccine is incubated in chick embryos. Viruses, being made up of purely genetic material, are prone to the process of "jumping genes" whereby the viruses may incorporate genetic material from the animal tissues in which they are incubated and subsequently introduce this material into the child receiving the vaccine. In theory, this could set the stage for later immune disorders including autoimmune diseases.[11-13]

3. Live virus vaccines subject to viral contamination:

Special concern for viral contamination is justified for the oral polio vaccine, which is incubated in monkey kidneys. African monkeys are now known to carry simian immunodeficiency viruses (SIVs), and it is now generally accepted that some mutation of one of the varieties of SIVs was the original source of the AIDS epidemic. In 1985, a SIV was discovered very similar to the AIDS virus. This, together with the fact that the earliest known cases of AIDS were near in time and location to the polio vaccine programs in Africa, raises the question whether the polio vaccine, possibly contaminated with the SIV, could have been the original source for AIDS.

Articles have appeared reviewing this matter and calling for further research.[14,15] Although polio vaccines are now screened for the AIDS virus, the question is more academic. New SIVs continue to be discovered, so that there still exists the possibility of viral contamination.

4. Interactions of the immune and nervous systems:

If childhood vaccines are capable of bringing about derangements of the immune system by mechanisms outlined above, it is probable that they may in some instances bring about comparable disturbances of the brain and nervous system. Hugh H. Fudenberg, MD, considered by many to be one of the leading immunologists of our times, has pointed out that there is a uniquely close association between the nervous system and the immune system with many cell receptors common to both systems.[16] If immunologic injuries are brought about by vaccines, it is reasonable to assume that they may at times be transferred to the brain and nervous system, this, in turn, can result in various forms of neurobehavioral problems.[17]

5. Interference with natural processes:

In earlier times, measles, mumps, and rubella (German measles) were referred to as minor childhood diseases because, in the vast majority of instances, children passed through these illnesses without serious complications. Could it be that these minor childhood diseases were friends in disguise, compelling the immune system through struggle and exercise to become strong and better able to defend the body? At least one authority thinks so.

In Great Britain, there was a sharp increase in Crohn's disease, a potentially serious intestinal disorder, among children of East Indian origin who had been raised in Britain and therefore had been immunized with the MMR vaccine. In contrast, Crohn's disease remains rare in India where vaccines are not widely administered. Dr. John Walker-Smith of St. Bartholomew's Hospital in London, a specialist in intestinal diseases of children, offered the following concept:

> It is possible that the decline of many childhood infections might allow children in the West to grow up without the vigorous development of their immune systems that such infections would ordinarily promote.
> One wonders whether that stimulation of the immune system, particularly in early childhood, may be advantageous in later life.[18]

A survey reviewed in Lancet (34:1071-1074) reported a 3.01 increased risk of Crohn's disease and a 2.53 increased risk of ulcerative colitis in people who had received the measles vaccine compared with unvaccinated people. The authors concluded that the measles vaccine may play a role in development of Crohn's disease and ulcerative colitis.

It is true that there were occasional serious complications from these diseases. For instance, measles in former times was complicated by encephalitis in one out of every 1,000 or 2,000 cases, sometimes leading to blindness, deafness, or death. If we take a position against the MMR vaccine, does this mean we accept these occasional complications? By no means. Good nutrition and a clean environment are highly protective against the serious complications. In Third World countries, high doses of vitamin A over short periods of time have been found to be protective with marked reduction of complications.[19]

There may be other answers.

A rational position about the MMR vaccine would be this: If it is found to cause more serious diseases than it is preventing - and there are many reasons for believing this is the case - then other answers should be sought.

6. The Pertussis (whooping cough) vaccine, surrounded by controversy

In a 1990 medical report it was stated that, throughout the world, pertussis remains a major cause of morbidity and mortality among infants, with an estimated 600,000 deaths annually.[20] Because of fear of a return of pertussis epidemics, the pertussis vaccine is one of the most strongly supported measures by public health services in the United States, but it is also one of the most controversial.

The seldom publicized history of the pertussis vaccine in Sweden, gives an entirely different point of view from that of the US public health service. Sweden banned the pertussis vaccine in 1979, and yet Sweden now has the second lowest infant mortality rate in the world, whereas the United States ranks a very poor 20th. or lower.

During the 1970s in Sweden, despite general pertussis immunization, pertussis returned after more than ten years of absence.[21] The disease became endemic. Surveys showed that 84% of children with pertussis had been fully vaccinated against the disease. Concluding that the pertussis vaccine was ineffective, it was banned in 1979. Subsequently, the incidence of the disease gradually increased, but deaths remained rare. One authority concluded that the disease is now much milder than in earlier times as an explanation for the very low death rate.

In conformance with this outlook, a report in 1984 stated that the pertussis mortality was generally very low in industrialized countries and there was no difference in severity and incidence of pertussis between countries with high, low and zero immunizations rates.[22]

Earlier it was stated that the pertussis vaccine had been the most controversial among childhood vaccines. Briefly summarized in the following are some of the reasons:

- A 1994 survey published in *the Journal of the American Medical Association* reported that children receiving pertussis vaccine were about six times more likely to develop asthma than those not receiving the vaccine.[23]

- In 1974, Japan raised the age of pertussis vaccination to two years of age, rather than giving it during early infancy as is done in the United States. Since that time, there has been a decline in sudden infant deaths (cot deaths) and spinal meningitis among Japanese infants. In spite of the lack of pertussis vaccine for infants, Japan is credited with one of the lowest infant morality rates in the world.[24]

- In *the Journal of Infectious Diseases* in 1992 there was a report of the DPT vaccine (diphtheria-pertussis-tetanus) provoking a significantly higher incidence of paralytic poliomyelitis in Oman during a polio epidemic in that country.[25] This report can be interpreted to indicate that the DPT vaccine can lower the resistance of the vaccinated child, opening the way for other diseases. Although the wild polio virus does not exist in the United States at this time, the counterpart in this country may be the increasing incidence of common respiratory infections, asthma and other forms of allergies, and a variety of neurobehavioral disorders.

- Perhaps the greatest source of controversy for the pertussis vaccine has been its implication in causing brain damage and various stages of autism among vaccinated children. A number of medical publications by defenders of the pertussis vaccine have attempted to dismiss this causal relationship, such as one recently issued in the *Journal of the American Medical Association*.[20] However, many would question the validity of this study which was limited to seven days. It did not take into account the possibility of delayed reactions, which may far outnumber acute reactions taking place within seven days. In the case of cancer we know that there may be a delay of many years between the original insult and onset of cancer, and this may be the case for brain injuries following vaccines. For this reason the true incidence of brain damage and autism from vaccines may be much greater than officially recognized.

- In a survey of a pertussis epidemic in Cincinnati in 1993 it was found that from 74% to 82% of children contracting pertussis had been highly immunized.[26] Although different interpretations were given by the authors, it would appear that this report corroborates conclusions in Sweden that the vaccine is ineffective.

7. *Chronic fatigue immune dysfunction syndrome* (CFIDS) *and childhood vaccinations*

CFIDS is a disease which afflicts young adults, predominantly women. It may be more than coincidental that the affected age groups, primarily in their twenties and thirties, are those in which childhood immunizations began to take momentum.

Immunologic abnormalities found in patients with CFIDS include an abnormal activation of the immune system and a decrease in uncommitted immune cells.[4,27] As previously mentioned, lymphocytes are a class of white blood cells that govern the immune system. These are divided into T-helper cells, which act as accelerators for the immune system, and T-suppressor cells, which act as brakes to reduce responses. In health, these two systems are perfectly balanced. In CFIDS, the T-helper cells are supercharged, turning out excessive immune proteins long after the threat is over. One of these is interleukin-2, usually excessively elevated in CFIDS patients.[27] The T-helper cells, in turn, are subdivided into "memory cells," which have been committed to previous challenges such as viruses, bacteria, or vaccines. Once committed, the memory cells are incapable of responding to new challenges. The second type of T-helper cells is the "naive cell" which serves as a reservoir for responses to new infectious or antigenic invasions. The key finding in CFIDS patients is a measurable shift in balance with increase in memory cells and decrease in naive cells.[4]

Undoubtedly this sounds complicated to those unfamiliar with these terms, but the interpretation is simple. The increase in interleukin-2 and memory cells indicates that the immune system has been over stimulated and overtaxed; the decrease in naive cells, which is necessary for new infectious challenges, means that the body is less able to defend itself. These are precisely the changes that could be predicted from childhood immunizations in their present forms and schedules. It would be highly interesting to do these tests on children after vaccinations, of course following standard scientific protocols. If it were found there are similar changes to those now being identified in CFIDS patients, then childhood vaccinations must be implicated as a predisposing cause of CFIDS.

Conclusions:

All of the foregoing discussion leads to one basic question: Does society, through the agency of government, have the right to compel parents to vaccinate their children against their (the parents') wishes? Although still a minority, there does appear to be an increasing number of parents who are militantly opposed to vaccines for their children.

The proponents of compulsory or mandated vaccines take the position that, if vaccines are made optional to all parents, the level of mass immunizations may fall to the point where epidemics of former times may return. On the surface this is a compelling argument. On the other hand, there is the moral issue: Of all human rights, the right of free choice as to what happens to our bodies or the choice of parents as to what is done to the bodies of their children should be one of the most sacred and inviolable. How do we reconcile these two viewpoints?

I believe that both viewpoints, that of safety and restoration of human rights, will be best served by granting parents perfect freedom to accept or reject immunizations for their children as they see fit. Growing numbers of people believe that vaccine programs have not been adequately researched to determine their long-term safety. As long as parents have the option of rejecting vaccines for their children, they have it in their power to compel technologic advances that would bring greater safety in the field. On the other hand, if current vaccination programs become universally mandated, a process already far advanced, in my opinion, the inevitable result would be scientific stagnation and a perpetuation of the dangers listed above.

References

1. Fitzgerald S, Jaffe M. Asthma death rate is up in Philadelphia. *Philadelphia Inquirer*. December 8, 1994:2,A22.

2. *The Human Ecologist*.(National HEAL). Fall 1992 (#55):6.

3. *Health Care & A Child's Ability To Learn; A Survey of Elementary School Teachers*. American Academy of Pediatrics (with the National PTA). September 1992.

4. *News from* NIAID (National Institute of Allergy and Infectious Disease). Washington, DC:National Institutes of Health, Laurie K. Doepel, February 3, 1993.

5. Miller N. *Vaccines: Are They Really Safe and Effective?* (A Parent's Guide to Childhood Shots). Santa Fe, NM:New Atlantean Press; 1992.

6. Scheibner V. *Vaccination; 100 Years of Orthodox Research Shows That Vaccines Represent a Medical Assault on the Immune System*. Santa Fe, NM:New Atlantean Press; 1993.

7. Coulter HL, Fisher BL. A *Shot in the Dark*. Garden City Park, NY: Avery Publishing Group; 1991.

8. Brody JA, McAlister R. Depression of tuberculin sensitivity following measles vaccination *Am Rev Respir Dis* 1996;90:607-611.

9. Brody JA, et al. Depression of the tuberculin reaction by viral vaccines. *N Engl J Med*. 1964;271:1294-1296.

10. Eibl M, et al. Abnormal T-lymphocyte subpopulations in healthy subjects after tetanus booster immunization. *N Eng J Med*. 1984;310(3):198-199 Letter.

11. Singer S. *Human Genetics*. New York:Freemand and Company; 103.

12. Blanck G, et al. Multiple insertions and tandem repeats of Origin-Mins Simian virus 40 DNA in transformed rat and mouse cells. J Virol. May 1988:1520-1523.

13. Kumar S, Miller LK. Effects of serial passage of Autographa Californica nuclear polyhidroses virus in cell culture. Virus Research.1987; 7:335-349.

14. Kyle SW. Simian retroviruses, polio vaccine, and the origin of AIDS. Lancet. 1992;339:601-602.

15. Martin B. Polio vaccines and the origin of AIDS: the career of a threatening idea. Townsend Letter for Doctors. January 1994;97-100.

16. Singh VK, Fudenberg HH. Can blood immunocytes be used to study neuropsychiatric disorders? J Clin Psychiatry. 1986;47(12):592-595.

17. Coulter HL. Vaccination, Social Violence, and Criminality. Berkeley, CA:North Atlantic Books; 1990.

18. Schmeck H, Jr. Baffling rise of intestinal disorder in the young. New York Times HEALTH. December 1988.

19. Hussey GD. A randomized trial of vitamin A in children with severe measles. N Engl J Med. 1990;323:160-164.

20. Gale JL, et al. Risk of serious acute neurological illness after immunization with diphtheria-pertussis-tetanus vaccine. JAMA. 1994;271(1):37-41.

21. Scheibner V. Vaccination; 100 Years of Orthodox Research Shows That Vaccines Represent a Medical Assault on the Immune System. Santa Fe, NM:New Atlantean Press; 1993:33-46.

22. Trollfors B. Bordetella pertussis whole cell vaccines: efficacy and toxicity. Acta Paediatr Scand. 1984;73:417-425.

23. Odent MR, et al. Pertussis vaccination and asthma: is there a link? JAMA. 1994;272(8):592-593 Letter.

24. Scheibner V. Vaccination; 100 Years of Orthodox Research Shows That Vaccines Represent a Medical Assault on the Immune System. Santa Fe, NM:New Atlantean Press; 1993:35-49.

25. Sutter RW, et al. Attributable risk of DTP (diphtheria-tetanus-pertussis) injection in provoking paralytic poliomyelitis during a large outbreak in Oman. J Infect Dis. 1992;165:444-449.

26. Miller, MW. Efficacy of whooping-cough vaccines is questioned by latest research data. Wall Street J, July 7, 1994.

27. Chaney PR. Interleukin-2 and the chronic fatigue syndrome. Ann Intern Med. 1989;110(4):321.

CHAPTER 12
Multiple chemical sensitivity: causes, mechanisms and treatment

In its advanced stages, patients with multiple chemical sensitivities (MCS) must live in the proverbial "glass house" which must remain virtually free of air-borne or fugitive chemicals. For these sufferers, even traces of vapors from perfumes, petrochemicals, cleaning solutions, tobacco smoke, paints, varnishes, and many other commercial products can cause illness. Chemical odors which an ordinary person would scarcely notice can be incapacitating to patients with MCS. Considering that MCS is poorly understood and its very existence questioned by some medical authorities, the lot of MCS patients is often singularly lonely and difficult.

Although MCS remains controversial at some levels, this syndrome is now recognized as a disease by several federal agencies including The Social Security Administration, the Department of Housing and

Urban Development, and in the Americans with Disability Act of July 26, 1990. It has been the object of intense Congressional interest and investigation as a result of large numbers of veterans from the Persian Gulf conflict returning with many symptoms consistent with MCS syndrome.

What are the causes of multiple chemical sensitivity?

The prime cause of MCS must be attributed to the massive increase in private and public use of volatile organic compounds (VOCs) in the past 50 years. VOCs have several unique characteristics. They tend to be volatile and escape into the air as fugitive chemicals. Being lipid or fat soluble, they have an affinity for the lipid tissues of the body. The brain is a prime target because of its high lipid content and rich blood supply. Cell membranes, being largely made up of lipids, are also subject to attack.

Before World War II, less than one billion pounds per year of volatile organic compounds were produced by the United States. By 1976, production had soared to 163 billion pounds per year,[1] confirming the prevalence of these chemicals. A study of 400 residents of New Jersey, North Dakota, and North Carolina found traces of up to 10 volatile organic compounds in exhaled breaths of the subjects.[1]

The increasing stress on energy efficiency in modern buildings combined with increasing use of commercial chemicals stand as the prime causes of MCS.

The mechanism for multiple chemical sensitivity?

The liver has been referred to as the chemical factory of the body. One of the offices of the liver is that of chemical detoxification. Although the process is complicated, the detoxification process is centered around two enzyme systems.

The first is centered around an enzyme system called cytochrome oxidase P450. This enzyme converts (by an *oxidative process*) the lipid-soluble state of volatile organic compounds into a more water-soluble form, in which they can be more readily excreted by the kidneys.

There is an adverse side to this process in that the water-soluble forms of the VOCs may be more toxic than their parent compounds.

If the second phase of detoxification, *conjugation*, does not keep pace with the increased volume of VOCs processed by the first, oxidative phase, the result may be heightened toxicity.

Nature never designed these enzyme systems to process the massive burden of volatile organic compounds with which they are now commonly confronted. There is evidence that the P450 system becomes weakened in patients with Multiple Chemical Sensitivity,[2,3] as a result of prolonged exposures or a single massive exposure to VOCs. By a process of "suicide inactivation," these enzymes may become progressively weakened and crippled by toxic exposures so the liver is less able to clear these chemicals from the system.

The age at which exposures take place is an important consideration. It has been estimated that children and fetuses are up to 10 times more vulnerable to toxic chemicals than adults.[4,5] It is increasingly common for environmental physicians to see children with MCS, and unless current exposure levels to volatile organic compounds are rapidly reduced, this pattern is bound to increase.

Frequency of multiple chemical sensitivity

MCS was reviewed on a recent television program entitled "The Nature of Things: Allergies, Nothing to Sneeze At." The host of the program, David Suzuki, reported on his investigations of environmental illness. Some environmental centers, according to Suzuki, estimate that 30 million North Americans suffer from some degree of chemical sensitivity. Of these, 1% develop intolerance to virtually all chemicals.

Diagnosis of multiple chemical sensitivity

Two types of studies are useful in confirming MCS in patients exposed to such chemicals as pesticides and/or solvent vapors.

The first is the triple-headed SPECT brain scan, which involves the intravenous injection of radioactive glucose. This is taken up by the brain and photographed by scintigraphy.

A research study, with sponsors including the US

Department of Health and Human Services, found that SPECT scans of patients exposed to neurotoxic chemicals indicated a "random thinning of cortical gray matter" (tissue in the cortex of the brain).[6]

The authors of the study concluded that symptomatic patients with a history of chemical exposures had significantly diminished cerebral blood flow and that "significant impairment of brain function may last for years after exposure to neurotoxic chemicals has ceased."

The second approach is to evaluate patients with MCS for disorders of porphyrin metabolism. Because many patients with MCS demonstrate neuropsychiatric symptoms similar to the porphyrias, well over 50% of patients with MCS have been found to have abnormal porphyrin tests in pilot studies. One such study is now being conducted at the Mayo Clinic in Rochester, Minnesota, not yet published.

Treatment of multiple chemical sensitivity

It may be just an educated guess, but it is probably not far from wrong to say 90% of treatment of MCS is the avoidance of fugitive chemicals. Much like radiation, the adverse effects of chemical exposures are probably cumulative. Once the process of chemical sensitization begins, each additional exposure may result in further cascading of the problem.

In our experience, many employees who became ill with MCS due to occupational chemical exposure may lead perfectly normal and active lives in controlled conditions where fugitive VOCs are absent or minimal. However, if and when they attempt to return to former conditions in the workplace, they quickly become ill again.

This raises a very interesting question: Why don't we clean up schools and the workplaces to a level of air purity that can be tolerated by patients with MCS? These unfortunates may be thought of as the miners' canaries. The canaries, being more sensitive to toxic gases, quickly died when gases escaped into the mines, thus warning the miners of danger. Patients with MCS may serve the same warning role for the rest of us. Unless we clean up indoor environments to a level of safety that they can tolerate, there may be many more victims.

Additional treatments include the antioxidant vitamins (vitamins E and C and beta carotene), chemical-free and pesticide-free foods, and other nutritive measures to enhance the detoxification pathways of the body. Some centers use intensive sauna programs for detoxification. Patients may do something similar by taking Epsom salt baths at home. However, this should be done cautiously, and under professional supervision.

If there is significant illness from chemical exposures, treatments should not be attempted without professional supervision.

References

1. *Multiple Chemical Sensitivities.* Washington, DC:National Research Council, National Academy Press; 1989:52.

2. Rea WJ. *Chemical Sensitivity. Vol I.* Boca Raton, FL: Lewis Publishers; 1993;65: 71-73.

3. Beaune P, et al. Autoantibodies against cytochrome P450; role in human disease. *Adv Pharmacol.* 1994;30:199-245. (Note: *This article uses the term "suicide inactivation" as a mechanism whereby foreign chemicals may damage and deactivate the P450 enzyme system.*)

4. *Pesticides in Diets of Infants and Children.* Washington, DC: National Research Council, National Academy Press; 1993:3.

5. *Neurotoxicity: Identifying and Controlling Poisons of the Nervous System.* Washington, DC:Superintendent of Documents, Government Printing Office; April 1990:49. GPO Stock #052-003-01184-1.

6. Heuser G, Mens I, Alarrios F. NeuroSPECT findings in patients exposed to neurotoxic chemicals. *Toxicol Industr Health.* 1994 (4/8):861-871.

Recommended reading

Ashford NA, Miller CS. *Chemical Exposures, Low Levels, and High Stakes.* New York:Van Nostrand Reinhold;1991.

Multiple Chemical Sensitivities. Washington, DC: National Research Council, National Academy Press; 1992.

Rea WJ. *Chemical Sensitivity. Vol I, II and III.* Boca Raton, FL: Lewis Publishers; Vol I, 1992; Vol II, 1994, Vol.III, 1995 .

CHAPTER 13

Combined exposures to multiple chemicals may greatly enhance their toxicity

Much of the current complacency about human chemical exposures is due to the method of toxicity testing, based on animal studies, in which a single chemical is tested to find an estimated "safe" level for human exposure.[1] Such testing is mandated by the Delaney Amendment of 1958 which requires the testing of potentially toxic chemicals for carcinogenic properties. There are several flaws and inadequacies in this system,[2,3] but perhaps the greatest flaw is that it does not take into account the effects of simultaneous human exposures to multiple environmental chemicals and their additive effects. We have previously mentioned the study in which 10 volatile chemicals were collected from the breath, indoor air, outdoor air and drinking water of 400 residents of New Jersey, North Carolina and North Dakota.[4]

Considering the technical difficulties and expense of testing even one chemical, it is partly understandable why the testing of a vast variety of chemical combinations has not been required by our present laws. However, three recent publications point to the feasibility, as well as the urgent need for more such studies and reevaluation of our safety standards in this area.[5-7]

In our first example, an outbreak of three sick building syndromes (SBS) in two high schools and the Federal Department of Justice building in Washington DC led researchers from Georgetown University Medical Center and the National Institutes of Health to conclude that chronic fatigue syndrome is often associated with SBS. The symptoms of affected people included headaches, fatigue, muscle pains, rhinitis, sinusitis, memory problems, low-grade fevers, eye irritation, and sensitivity to light. No single chemical was found above established safety levels. No viral or biologic agent was found. The authors suggested that the cause may have been low levels of contaminants acting "in concert," or synergistically to produce overlapping syndromes.[5]

The second example involved a study of environmental chemicals which are estrogenic; that is, they simulate the effects of the female hormone, estrogen, in the human body. The three chemicals studied (dieldrin, endosulfan and toxaphene) were too weak to affect biological systems when tested singly, but in combination, two of these chemicals were a thousand times more potent than either alone in their estrogenic effects.[6] The authors suggested such combinations may pose a risk for breast cancer and decrease human semen quality.

The final example concerns the Persian Gulf War Syndrome, a subject of historical as well as human and scientific interest. Of the three-quarters of a million service personnel involved in the Persian Gulf War, approximately 30,000 have complained of neurologic (nervous system) symptoms of unknown etiology. The study, which was performed on hens, involved three chemicals: the anti-nerve agent pyridostigmine bromide, which was given to some personnel, the insecticide permethrin, and an insect repellent applied to the skin. The toxic effects of each agent alone was minimal, but a combination of all three often led to severe neurologic damage. The authors postulated that the pyridostigmine bromide, which inhibits detoxification enzymes in the body, may have led to greater concentrations of the other two chemicals, both of which are potentially neurotoxic, to reach the nervous system.[7]

In the scientific realm these studies properly will be considered preliminary, and more studies will be called for. But studies take time, and time is running out for our children. In the final analysis, it is the parents who must protect the children.

References

1. Pesticides in Diets of Infants and Children. Washington DC: National Research Council; 1993:123-157.

2. Pesticides in Diets of Infants and Children. Washington DC: National Research Council; 1993:3

3. Mott L, Snyder K. Pesticide Alert. San Francisco: National Resources Defense Council, Sierra Club Books; 1987.

4. Wallace LA et al. The TEAM study: personal exposures to toxic substances in air, drinking water, and breath of 400 residents of New Jersey, North Carolina and North Dakota. Environ. Research 43:290-307.

5. Chester AC, Levine PH. Concurrent sick building syndrome and chronic fatigue syndrome: epidemic neuromyasthenia revised. Clinical Infectious Diseases 18 (Suppl 1):1996:S43-S48.

6. Arnold SF, et al. Synergistic activation of estrogen receptor with combinations of environmental chemicals. Science. 1996;272;1489-1492.

7. Abou-Donia MB, et al. Neurotoxicity resulting from coexposure to pyridostigmine bromide, DEET, and permitrin: implications of Gulf war chemical exposures. J Tox & Environ Health. 1996;48:35-56.

CHAPTER 14
Food allergies and childhood behavior

The subject of food allergies has been controversial in the medical field. Conventional wisdom holds that food allergies are relatively unimportant in health problems of children, the exception being the relatively infrequent instances when children break out in hives or some other allergic manifestation immediately after ingesting an offending food (technically known as Type I allergic reaction).

Other physicians, predominantly those schooled in the field of environmental medicine, believe that food allergy problems are relatively common. They may manifest as delayed reactions in many forms including asthma, hay fever, eczema, irritable bowel, seizures, headaches, behavioral problems, hyperactivity, and some forms of mental illness.

Probably the single more important study confirming the widespread role of food allergies in childhood health problems was conducted by Joseph Egger, MD, of Munich, Germany.[1] The study involved

76 children specially selected because of severe hyperactivity and behavioral problems, as well as a high proportion with other problems including headaches, abdominal pains, and seizures. In the study, the children were placed on an "oligoantigenic diet" from which all foods with high allergic potential were removed from the diet. The restrictive diet was continued for several weeks during which time 82% of the children showed significant improvement in behavioral problems and hyperactivity. Most of the associated symptoms (headaches, abdominal pains, and seizures) improved as well. Previously eliminated foods were reintroduced after several weeks, one at a time in intervals as long as five days. In this way offending foods were identified by reappearance of symptoms. It should be noted that reactions were often delayed two or three days after reintroduction of the allergy-causing food, proving the prevalence of delayed-type reactions (Type IV allergic reaction).

A well-designed study at Cornell Medical Center, Manhasset, New York, has confirmed that "foods and additives are common causes of the attention deficit hyperactive disorder in children.[2]"

One of the better known figures in food allergies is the pediatric allergist, Doris Rapp, MD of Buffalo, New York. Dr. Rapp has been a frequent guest on popular television shows where she has shown videos made in her office of hyperactive children during treatment. In these demonstrations, the child would be given sublingual (under the tongue) drops containing extracts of a food which, by previous testing, had been found to be offending to the child. The child then went into wild, uncontrolled behavior until neutralization drops were administered, also based on previous testing. The child then returned to normal behavior. As explained by Dr. Rapp, this Jekyll-Hyde behavior could be turned on and off, almost like a light switch, by administering the offending food, followed by sublingual neutralization. It should be mentioned that this pattern has been confirmed by double-blind studies in her office.

As with other types of allergies, the incidence of food allergies appears to be increasing in children. The causes appear to be chemical in nature. Patients with multiple chemical sensitivities, the result of volatile organic compound exposures, usually have digestive impairments. These are caused by damage to intestinal mucous membranes by the volatile organic compounds.[3]

Chemical food additives may also play a role. As a result of this mucosal damage there may be increased intestinal permeability with large-scale leakage of incompletely digested food molecules into the bloodstream. These food molecules are foreign to the human system and, therefore, are prone to induce allergies and sensitization. This, in lay terms, is the probable explanation for the increasing incidence of food allergies.

The digestive process is regulated by an intestinal immune system (the secretory IgA system).[4-11] This immune system, sometimes referred to as "antiseptic paint," coats the surface of intestinal mucosa. The secretory IgA antibodies work by adhering to undigested food particles and preventing their absorption before digestion is complete. It is a system of almost inconceivable intelligence, because each food particle of untold billions of food particles must be recognized and intercepted in this way. In Chapter 10, it was pointed out that many published studies show the suppressive effects of antibiotics on the systemic immune system. Although we are not aware of comparable studies of antibiotics on the intestinal system, it can be safely assumed that antibiotics have the same suppressive effects here, thus also contributing to "the leaky gut" or increased intestinal permeability.

Several options are available in identifying offending allergenic foods in an individual. The first and perhaps the best is the elimination-rechallenge diet. Guidelines for this diet are provided in Dr. Doris Rapp's books (listed at the end of this chapter). It is conducted in the home. Its success, however, depends on rigid control of the diet during the elimination and reintroduction phases. Problems commonly arise when the child is visiting with friends or when at school where the youngster may be able to obtain unauthorized foods.

Another approach to identifying problem foods is blood testing. There are several types performed by physicians. Finally, there are skin tests, commonly done by physicians whose practices include treatment of allergy.

Treatment depends on the severity of the food allergy. In milder cases, the elimination of several of the major offending foods from the diet, once they have been identified, may be sufficient to relieve symptoms. More serious cases may require further measures. In addition to removing the worst of the problem foods from the diet, a four-day rotation diet may be beneficial, where a given food is not eaten more than one out of four days. In the field of environmental medicine, sublingual food neutralization drops may go far in relieving symptoms. Neutralization doses are determined by skin tests using the technique of serial dilution titration, in which differing dilutions of a given food extract are injected into the skin to find which dilution first gives a skin reaction. This is then used to determine the "neutralizing dose." Experience has shown that a majority of children are significantly helped by these drops. When they fail, as they sometimes do, other causes must be sought.

Note: Guidelines for the rotating diet are found in the books of Dr. Doris Rapp *(see end of chapter).*

Breast feeding an infant will go far in protecting against allergies. Maternal milk contains antibodies and other factors that cannot be reproduced in infant formulas.

References

1. Egger J, et al. Controlled trial of oligoantigenic diet treatment in the hyperkinetic syndrome. *Lancet.* 1984:540-545.

2. Boris M, Mandel FS. Foods and additives are common causes of the attention deficit hyperactive disorder in children. *Ann Allergy.* 1994;72:462-468.

3. Finn R. Interaction between allergy and chemical sensitivity. *Environ Med.* 1991;8(3):92-95.

4. Walker WA. Antigen absorption from the small intestine and gastrointestinal disease. *Pediatr Clin North Am.* 1975;22:713-746.

5. Walker WA, Hong R. Immunology of the gastro intestinal tract. Part 1. *J Pediatr.* 1973;83:517-530.

6. Walker WA, Wu M, Isselbacher KJ, Bloch KJ. Intestinal uptake of macromolecules, III, studies on the mechanism by which immunization interferes with antigen uptake. *J Immunol.* 1975;115:854-861.

7. Walker WA. Antigen handling by the gut. *Arch Dis Child.* 1978;53:527-531.

8. Walker WA, Isselbacher KJ. Uptake and transport of macromolecules by the intestine, possible role in clinical disorders. *Gastroenterology.* 1974;67:531-550.

9. Walker WA, et al. Intestinal uptake of macromolecules, IV, the effect of pancreatic duct ligation on the breakdown of antigen and antigen-antibody complexes on the intestinal surface. *Gastroenterology.* 1975;69:1223-1229.

10. Goldstine GB, Heiner DC. Clinical and immunological perspectives in food sensitivity, a review. *J Allergy.* 1970;46:270-291.

11. Tomasi TB Jr. Secretory immunoglobulins. N Engl J Med. 1972;287:500-506.

Recommended reading for parents

Rapp D. Is This Your Child? (Discovering and Treating Unrecognized Allergies). New York: William Morris and Company; 1991. (Available from Practical Allergy Research Foundation PO Box 60, Buffalo, NY 14223-0060, (716-875-0398 or 800-787-8780).

Rapp D, Bamberg D. The Impossible Child, in School - at Home. Buffalo,NY: Practical Allegy Research Foundation. 1986.

Rapp D. Is This Your Child's World? New York NY. Bantam. 1996 (716-875-0398)

Recommended reading for professionals

Brostoff J, Challacome SJ, ed. Food Allergy and Intolerance. London: Bailliere Tindall; 1987.

CHAPTER 15
Prenatal influences:

This chapter is reproduced from the book, **For Tomorrow's Children, A Manual for Future Parents,** *available from Foresight America, 5724 Clymer Road, Quakertown, Pa 18951*

Effects of the mother's thoughts and emotions during pregnancy on the baby-to-be

Nowhere is the time-honored adage, "thoughts are things," more true than during the course of pregnancy, a creative period in which the baby-to-be is highly plastic or malleable to the thoughts and emotions of the mother. History abounds with examples that show that imprints of the mother's thoughts and deeply held feelings may later manifest, for good or for ill, as personality traits, inclinations, and talents in the offspring.

The first authentic work on this subject was published in 1902 by R. Swinburne Clymer, MD: *Prenatal Culture.* The book did not offer scientific evidence to validate the subject, but it did present the concept in clear language and provided much philosophical support for its acceptance. The text was recently republished and must be considered the classic work on this intriguing subject.

Prenatal testing

Many cast a skeptical eye on the concept of prenatal influence. Instances of probable prenatal influences, no matter how numerous or convincing, are dismissed as anecdotal, because there is no way they can meet the standard of the double blind study, the procedure that has become the accepted standard of scientific proof. The double blind study is valid in the study of drugs and chemicals, but it doesn't lend itself to our present subject. For this reason we must resort to other forms of analysis and testing. For that reason, we must resort to other forms of testing and analysis.

Such testing is being done, which should meet the most stringent criteria of scientific standards. An organization, the Pre- and Peri-Natal Psychology Association of North America (PPPANA), has been formed by psychiatrists and psychologists to study prenatal influences, to document them in a scientific manner, and to publish their findings. This is being done in the quarterly journal, *Pre- and Peri-Natal Psychology Journal*, published by Human Sciences Press, Inc., 233 Spring Street, New York NY, 10013-1578.

One of the founding members of PPPANA,

Thomas Verny, MD, a psychiatrist in Toronto, Ontario, published a book, *The Secret Life of the Unborn Child*, in 1981. The book represents the first systematic study of prenatal influences with a review of published world literature dealing with the subject to that time. Some of the anecdotes cited in the book are fascinating and provocative.

One of the most striking stories is that of the Canadian Symphony Orchestra conductor, Boris Brott. On a radio program the interviewer asked how Brott became interested in music. After hesitating a moment, Brott replied, "You know, this may sound strange, but music has been a part of me since before birth." Somewhat puzzled, the interviewer asked him to explain.

"Well," said Brott, "as a young man, I was mystified by this unusual ability I had - to play certain pieces sight unseen. I'd be conducting a score for the first time and, suddenly, the cello line would jump out at me; I'd know the flow of the piece even before I turned the page of the score. One day I mentioned this to my mother, who is a professional cellist. I thought she'd be intrigued because it was always the cello line that was so distinct in my mind. She was; but when she heard what the pieces were, the mystery quickly solved itself. All the scores I knew sight unseen were ones she had played while she was pregnant with me."

Effect of stress on the unborn

Dr. Verny addressed the question of stress during

pregnancy and its potential effect on the fetus. He quoted from studies which showed that women subjected to severe and continuous stress during pregnancy tended to bear children with physical and emotional problems. But there were notable exceptions, depending on how the mother felt about her unborn child.

One striking example was given by Verny:

> It would be hard to imagine a more tumultuous pregnancy than the one a woman I'll call Susan endured. Husbandless - her spouse left her a few weeks after she learned she was expecting - and beset by constant financial problems, Susan had already encountered more than her share of difficulties when, in her sixth month, a precancerous cyst was found on one of her ovaries. Its immediate removal was urged, but when Susan was told that the required surgery would abort her child, she refused. In her mid thirties., Susan believed this was her last opportunity to have a child and she desperately wanted it. 'Nothing else mattered,' she told me later. 'I would have risked anything to have my baby.' On some level, I feel her child sensed that desire. Andrea, as the child was named, was born healthy and, at this writing, two years later, is a normal, happy, well-adjusted child.

In short, then, while the external stresses a woman faces matter, what matters most is the way she feels about her unborn child. Her thoughts and feelings are the material out of which the unborn child fashions himself. When they are positive and nurturing, the child can, as Andrea did, withstand shocks from almost any quarter. But the fetus cannot be misled either. If he is good at sensing what is on his mother's mind generally, he is even better at sensing her attitude towards him, as a group of ingeniously designed new psychologist studies show.

Dr. Verny cited a study of two thousand women followed through pregnancy and birth by Dr. Monika Lukesch, a psychologist at Constantine University in Frankfurt, West Germany. Dr. Lukesch concluded from her study that the mother's attitude had the single greatest effect on how an infant turned out. All her subjects were equally intelligent, and all had the same degree of prenatal care. The only major distinguishing factor was their attitudes towards their unborn children, and that turned out to have a critical effect on their infants. The children of accepting mothers, who looked forward to having a family, were much healthier, emotionally and physically, at birth and afterwards, than the offspring of the rejecting mothers.

The father's influence on the unborn

What about the father's influence? Dr. Verny said,

> All evidence indicates that the quality of a woman's relationship with her husband or partner - whether she feels happy and secure or, alternately, ignored and threatened - has a decisive effect on her unborn child. Dr. Lukesch, for example, rates the quality of a woman's relationship with her spouse second only to her attitude toward being a mother in determining the infant outcome.

Dr. Verny quoted another worker, Dr. Dennis Stott, who rated bad marriages or relationships as among the greatest causes of emotional and physical damage in the womb. According to Stott, even such widely recognized dangers as physical illness, smoking, and the performance of back-breaking labor during pregnancy pose less of a risk to the unborn child. He found unhappy marriages produced children who as babies were five times more fearful and jumpy than the offspring of happy relationships. At ages four and five, Dr. Stott found them to be undersized, timid, and emotionally dependent on their mothers to an inordinate degree.

Dr. Verny observed,

> It is also important to remember that a strong, nurturing mother-child bond can protect the fetus against even these very traumatic shocks.

Evidence of prenatal influence

The spring of 1989 issue of the *Pre- and Peri-Natal Psychology Journal* included a series of carefully documented studies presenting irrefutable evidence of prenatal influences at varying levels. In the editorial to the issue, Dr. Verny wrote:

> The great majority of physicians, nurses, and psychologists simply do not believe that babies can feel, think, remember, or communicate. How do we get them to change their minds? Obviously, there is no simple answer to this question. The problem is that this need for scientific

proof, which the health professionals profess to seek, really camouflages a complex web of unconscious fears. The obstetricians of Vienna in the 1860s would not, could not, comprehend that they were responsible for spreading puerperal (childbed) fever by not washing their hands, and this drove Dr.Ignaz Semmelweiss to suicide. Today's health professionals once again resist what in a few years' time will be as much of a common sense notion as washing one's hands between patient examinations.

In a subsequent article, "The Scientific Basis of Pre- and Peri-natal Psychology, Part I," Dr. Verny provided an extensive review of human and animal studies showing prenatal learning.

In the animal studies, Marion Diamond, a neuroanatomist at the University of California at Berkeley, placed pregnant rats in an environment with mazes and toys. For rats, mazes and toys involve learning, much as schooling does for children. These are called "enriched" environments. Offspring of enriched animals were found to have larger brains than the progeny of the control parents who were raised in plain cages. The offspring of the enriched animals also had larger levels of neurotransmitters and increase in glial cells (connecting fibers between brain cells). Furthermore, each succeeding generation had larger brain cortices. As Verny expressed it, "the enriched get richer."

In human studies, Donald Shetler, a professor music education at the University of Rochester, has studied the effect of music during pregnancy on infant development. Shetler evaluates the musical response of newborns by looking at attention span and body movements. Later he measures the child's ability to imitate rhythms and vocal sounds and to manipulate such sound-making objects as small bells. The sessions in Shetler's classroom-a music laboratory of tiny xylophones, drums, and musical toys - were videotaped for later analysis.

Shetler reports that infants exposed to music while in the womb show "remarkable attention behaviors, imitate accurately sounds made by adults, and structure vocalization earlier than controls" (babies not subjected to music before birth). He believes that prenatal music may, in fact, give babies a head start.

Dr. Verny's studies include psychiatric and other aspects of prenatal and childhood care: What are a child's fears? expectations? How did they develop? What corrections are necessary? How can the unborn and newborn child be better prepared for life experiences? In focusing on causes of early childhood problems, his study forced him to look not only at the impressions a child receives as a fetus but also at the environment in which the child was conceived. These findings, in turn, led him to recognize that the most important time in a child's life is the period up to a year before he is conceived. During this time parents must sort out and work out their problems and prepare themselves for motherhood and fatherhood.

A mother's feelings

The fetus, during pregnancy, is a highly plastic being, molded in large measure by the thoughts and feelings of the mother. If these are of a positive nature, they may manifest in later life as a relatively healthy and well-adjusted individual with increased intelligence and talents. If of a negative nature, they may result in later mental and physical health problems.

The single most important factor is how the mother feels about the unborn baby. If it is an accepted and desired pregnancy, almost any adversity may be overcome for the well-being of the baby. If it is an unwanted or indifferent pregnancy, the reverse may obtain.

The second most important factor is the relationship of the mother with her husband. If this is warm and supportive, the results will tend to be favorable.

Life's stresses, no matter how great, need not have an adverse effect if the mother carries a warm and nurturing feeling for her unborn infant.

Heredity is of course important, but in some instances prenatal influences, combined with good health care, may outweigh heredity. It is an indisputable fact that many great persons throughout history have been born to humble parents with limited intellectual capacities.

CHAPTER 16
Health freedom in America

The history of America from our earliest colonial days up to the present, has been a succession of struggles for freedom. The current struggle for health freedom may in time be recorded as another milestone and precedent in our nation's history.

Probably transcending any other problem in America today is that of the deteriorating health of our children. Steadily increasing allergic, immunologic, and neurobehavioral problems are occurring on a scale unknown in earlier generations. Unless reversed, this adverse health trend threatens the future of our nation.

Leading research scientists as well as a large and growing portion of the public are coming to believe that the causes of the deteriorating health of American children include toxic environmental chemicals, chemical food additives, pesticide residues in foods, commercial processing and denaturing of foods, polluted water, fluoridation, overuse of antibiotics, and excessive use of drugs to the exclusion of more natural therapies. We would add the current mandatory childhood immunization programs as among the many threats to the health and well-being of children.

The problem is of momentous importance, not unlike other crises in our nation's history. Public discontent with our present health system exists on a vast scale. The public is not being adequately protected against toxic environmental chemicals. Chemical food additives are rarely, if ever, thoroughly tested for their safety. Our present health system, which is largely drug-dependent, is increasingly coercive.

Many foreign countries have traditions of natural healing in which natural therapies are fully legal and extensively used. In America, these therapies are banned and practitioners harassed. One is reminded of the era of alcoholic prohibition in America (1919 to 1933), a time characterized by gangsters and lawlessness. If the prohibition of alcohol with all of its evils did not work, will the prohibition of natural healing, with its many potentials for good, remain enforced?

The ultimate answer is to restore free enterprise and freedom-of-choice to our health system. This will go far toward defusing present tensions.

Finally, children are far more vulnerable to toxic chemicals and to the effects of drugs than adults. If we are to save a generation of children, and with them our future as a nation, positive changes must come about soon.

CHAPTER 17

Conclusions

Conscientious parents attempting to raise healthy children are confronted with major challenges under today's conditions. Here is a summary:

- Sources of volatile toxic chemicals which contaminate indoor air of homes should be removed. Problems of dust and mold may require attention. With grace and diplomacy, parents should also police the indoor air of schools and day-care centers for these contaminations.

- Attention should be paid to indoor lighting. The best source is natural daylight through adequate windows or full-spectrum fluorescent lights. Cool-white fluorescent lights are the worst light source due to their limited color spectrum. When feasible, a child should spend at least one hour daily out-of-doors.

- Food should be sought which is free from chemical additives or pesticide residues. Organic foods (foods grown without chemical fertilizers, herbicides, or pesticides) are highly desirable. Unfortunately, these are not always available, and they are generally more expensive and beyond the means of many young families. If such is the case, we advise fresh market produce and products that have not been commercially processed, soaking fruit and vegetables in water with a little added baking soda or vinegar and then rinsing to remove chemical residues. For most this will be adequate.

- Parents should learn to recognize the sources of toxic heavy metals (especially lead, cadmium antimony and mercury) contamination, and protect children from exposure.

- In spite of major efforts by public officials to improve the quality of public water supplies, chemical contamination remains a common and pervasive problem. Traces of multiple volatile organic compounds are frequently present. The cumulative effect of these multiple chemicals may be sufficient to adversely affect the child. Lead from plumbing systems may be found in older homes (its use in homes is now largely banned). Regarding fluoridation, extensive studies have been done which fail to confirm any reduction in dental caries from fluoridated water but instead suggest that it may act as a toxin on enzymes of the body. If tap water is found to be unsafe for these reasons, spring water in glass bottles may be purchased for drinking and cooking. As another alternative, commercial water filters which can be attached to the sink are available at reasonable cost.

- Leading physicians and researchers at major medical centers are decrying the overuse of antibiotics in treating minor childhood illnesses. As an alternative, parents should learn the use of a few, "natural" remedies for home use. We have found that intelligent use of these substances will get the child through a majority of minor illnesses without the need for antibiotics.

- Parents should be allowed freedom of choice in accepting or refusing current immunization programs for their children.

- Ideally, all pregnancies should be planned. All children should be wanted.

In our experience, many parents bringing their children to us have already done considerable study and investigation of health matters on their own . These parents may not require more than a fine-tuning of programs they have already set in motion, along with medical therapies as indicated.

For other parents, much of this information is entirely new,. Their first reaction is to feel overwhelmed by the seeming immensity of their tasks. For this latter group we advise simply to take one step at a time, setting priorities for the most immediate problem areas. If this is done, things usually fall into place, and however difficult things may seem, the ultimate health of the child may, in time ,be achieved.

To recapitulate - we live in difficult times, and none more difficult than for parents seeking the best for their children. However, we have this consolation: through our recorded history, every major human advancement has come about through crises and difficulties. It may be that our present difficulties may presage another advancement of the human family, unlike and beyond any that has taken place before.

APPENDIX I
Case reports of environmental illness

CASE REPORT 1

Janet

Janet (not her real name) was 9 years old when she was brought to our office by her mother. Janet was a precocious child, as related by the mother with undisguised pride. She was very bright when she entered kindergarten, receiving highest ratings among 80 children. This scholastic excellence continued during the first two grades, but in the third grade she began to have difficulties. Although she remained in the 99th percentile in mathematics, her reading comprehension slipped to 51%. When seen by an ophthalmologist, she was found to have visual perception and focusing problems.

Along with her visual problems and lowered grade averages she began having other symptoms including hives, headaches, stomach (abdominal) pains, general achiness, and other flu like symptoms.

One afternoon, the child came home extremely ill and reported to the mother that she began feeling badly in the gymnasium where she was having physical education class. On investigation, the mother found that this area had been sprayed on a monthly basis with a commonly used organophosphate pesticide; the previous spraying had taken place six days before the day the child experienced her illness. At this point, the mother began to suspect that there might have been a relation between the pesticide exposure and the child's other symptoms.

After hearing Janet's history, I told the mother that, in my opinion, it was highly probable that prolonged exposures to the pesticide were the cause of Janet's deteriorating health and lowered school performance, although it would be very difficult to prove the relationship. I had learned from the Environmental Protection Agency that pesticides may remain airborne from two to eight weeks after application. This being the case, monthly sprayings could result in almost continuous exposure of the students.

Subsequently, the parents transferred Janet to another school where pesticides were not used. Janet once again became a top honor student, although all of her old symptoms would return if exposed to pesticides or herbicides, as when playing on a soccer field treated with herbicides or on one occasion when she went into a pet store where there had been flea-dipping of the pets.

Comments:

A movement called Integrated Pest Management (IPM) is rapidly becoming accepted. Emphasis is placed upon the use of non chemical alternatives to pesticides. When chemicals must be used, they are chosen and applied in ways that are least hazardous to people, property, or the environment. IPM methods have been adopted in school districts in Pennsylvania, New Jersey, Maryland, Texas, California, and Toronto, Canada. IPM methods are successful and generally reduce costs. At the time of this writing, there is a bill before the Pennsylvania State Legislature that, if it is passed, will require the adoption of IPM by all school districts in the state. It is the first of its kind, as far as we are aware.

Recommended reading:

Pest Control in the School Environment: Adopting Integrated Pest Management. Washington, DC: United States Environmental Protection Agency, Office of Pesticide Programs; August 1993.

CASE REPORT 2
Bradley

Bradley (*Parents asked us to use his real name*) is an eight-year-old boy with a variety of health problems including seizure disorder, attention deficit disorder, primary speech and language disorder, multiple chemical sensitivities, multiple food allergies and nasal allergies. Several years ago, he was placed under the care of another physician who did testing for foods and inhalants (dust, mold, pollen, etc.). Based on the testing, six major offending foods were eliminated from the diet and the remaining foods were given on a rotating basis. Allergy neutralization therapy was instituted for inhalants.

Under this treatment program his speech began to improve (he had not talked until about age five years), and his formerly frequent ear and respiratory infections were eliminated. When his former physician passed away, Bradley came under our care, and we have continued the previous therapies. Medication for his seizure disorder is under the supervision of a neurologist.

According to the history provided by the parents, the boy is exquisitely sensitive to chemical odors such as perfumes, petrochemicals, tobacco smoke, paints, and cleaning solutions. Exposures to these and other chemicals, as observed by the parents, have at times brought on seizures and profound behavioral changes of an adverse nature.

The mother believes the seizures have been present since birth, although they were not diagnosed until some time later. It is important to note that the mother did work in a new office building with new carpets, copying machines, and other chemical exposures during her pregnancy with Bradley. Although speculative, his chemical sensitization and other health problems might be attributable to in-utero chemical exposures during this time.

Bradley's former physician authorized homebound schooling so as to avoid chemical exposures in the school, which the physician as well as the parents believed were injurious to the boy. At the present time, the school administration has issued a truancy charge and is moving to have the boy returned to school. The parents are appealing this charge so as to continue home schooling. The matter remains in the court. The parents are determined to do all they can to prevent Bradley from being placed back in the school environment.

Comments:

As reviewed in Chapter 12, chemical exposures can impair a child's ability to learn. If this is the case in otherwise healthy children, and there is much evidence that this commonly take place, the effects are manyfold greater in a child with chemical sensitivities. If there is a compulsory return of the boy to chemical exposures commonly present in modern buildings, in all likelihood this will bring about behavioral retrogression and a worsening of the seizure disorder.

This case exemplifies a common dilemma for schools and parents. In fairness to the school administration involved here, they are acting in a framework of general unawareness of the hazards of volatile chemical exposures, and they are under an obligation to fulfill the laws governing school attendance. However, the parents are acting under a higher obligation: that of protecting their child.

Pioneering environmental centers such as those in Dallas and Buffalo, New York,, have gone far in developing laboratory parameters for documenting chemical injury. These include blood tests that show a high percentage of abnormalities in chemically sensitive patients, abnormalities of lymphocyte subpopulations (lymphocytes are a form of white blood cell that govern the immune system), and abnormalities of other immune markers. Another test of paramount importance in chemically injured patients in the SPECT Scan of the brain. This involves the injection of radioactive glucose, which is taken up by the brain and photographed by scintigraphy. Pilot studies are showing reduced and irregular uptake in many chemically injured patients.[1]

There are several problems for the average family needing the tests for their children: the tests are expensive, they are often not covered by insurance, and they are often dismissed as "experimental." In other words, concerned parents are told that they must wait on the finer points of scientific documentation before taking measures to protect their children. Considering the high toll on children resulting from this inaction, can we afford to wait?

Reference:

1. Hauser G, Metta I, Alsmos F. NeuroSPECT findings in patients exposed to neurotoxic chemicals. *Toxicology and Industrial Health* 1994;10: 861-871.

Case Report 3
Donald

Donald ia a 13-year-old boy who has had asthma since early childhood, but in previous years his asthma had been relatively mild and controlled with minimal medication. In the beginning of a recent fall semester he was transferred to a school where the roof was being renovated After resumption of classes, large numbers of the student body and faculty became ill with complaints of difficulty breathing, headaches, nausea, and dizziness. Donald began having serious asthma attacks, which resulted in his missing nearly half of the school days during the next several months. Donald's mother, who provided most of the medical history, related that whenever he would attempt to return to school, invariably he developed an attack of asthma within one hour of entering the building.

Potential blame for the problem was placed on cement sealants, roofing tar, spray paints, and insulation adhesives, giving rise to solvent-type fumes that were sucked from the roof into the building through vents.

An environmental consulting firm was hired to check chemical levels in the indoor air. The air analysis did find a number of solvent-type chemicals, but the levels were judged to be far below the levels considered hazardous to human health according to currently accepted standards. The building was declared safe.

When Donald was brought to our office, we believed there was sufficient chemical evidence to necessitate his removal from the school and placement on homebound schooling for the remainder of the school year in spite of the negative report by the environmental firm.

Comments:

This case has several interesting and, we believe, instructive features. As reviewed in newspaper articles dealing with the school situation, no one seriously questioned that the symptoms and illnesses of students and faculty were real. Neither were there explanations for the seeming paradox that these illnesses occurred at levels of chemicals judged to be far below those that would be hazardous to human health.

The question resolves to one that has been plaguing the highest levels of researchers in environmental toxicity: What are the adverse effects of continued low levels of exposure to the multitudes of environmental chemicals which are known to be toxic at higher levels? This question appears repeatedly in the writings of the researchers.[1-4]

Standards of safety for solvent fumes are based on testing each chemical separately and not in combination with other chemicals. However, chemicals often do not come separately in modern buildings but in multitudes. For sake of argument, assume there are 10 or 15 solvent type fumes in a building, each at sufficiently low levels to be judged as safe. Would there be an additive effect of the 10 or 15 chemicals? Considering the technical difficulties of testing even one chemical, the difficulties of testing 10 or 15 chemicals in combination would be almost insurmountable.

One does not have to read far in the publications of authoritative research groups such as the National Research Council and the National Academy of Sciences to realize this is a foremost question on their minds and that they hold strong suspicions that this additive effect of chemicals may be a common phenomenon.[1]

In addition, current safety standards for "permissible exposure levels" for volatile organic chemicals are based on testings of healthy adults and do not make allowances for the greater vulnerability of children, estimated to be six to ten times greater than adults.

There is another question for which airborne solvents may hold the answer. Why has the incidence as well as the severity of asthma been steadily increasing in recent decades, especially among the younger generation? The national death rate from asthma has been reported to increase 46% between 1977 and 1991. Why this increase?

As pointed out in Chapter 5, the production of volatile organic compounds in the United States is estimated to have increased 163-fold in the past 50 or 60 years. As more energy-efficient buildings with less air circulation were built in the late 1970s, the levels of ambient chemicals in indoor air increased.

Volatile solvent-type chemicals have an affinity for the fatty tissues of the body. Cell membranes, being lipoprotein in nature, are subject to damaging attacks by the volatile chemicals. The mucous membranes of the respiratory tract are especially vulnerable to the solvent-containing air. In *The Journal of Environmental Medicine* (8;3:92), Ronald Finn, MD, of Liverpool, England, blamed the increasing incidence of allergies and asthma on "chemically induced surface mucosal damage which facilitates the entry of antigens" (dust, pollen, mold, etc.) through the damaged membranes.

Concluding remarks:

These three case reports have a common feature: Parents may have a truer insight into the nature of their children's ills than the authorities. Although the parents may be scientifically unlettered, the combination of common observation and parental instinct may come closer to the mark than the judgments of medical professionals..

One is reminded here of the case of Hungarian-born Ignaz Semmelweis. He received his medical degree in 1944 and was appointed a position at the obstetric clinic in Vienna where mortality rates ranged as high as 25% to 30%, largely from puerperal fever, a contagious disease. He Observed that death rates were highest on the student division where students would often go, without washing their hands, from the dissecting room to the delivery room. Semmelweis deduced that the students were carrying the contagion from infected persons to other patients. When Semmelweis instituted the practice of washing hands in chlorinated water between patients, the death rate fell dramatically to 1.27%. It should be remembered that this was a time before there was any understanding of infectious diseases or sanitation.

Although younger medical professionals recognized the significance of his discovery, the medical community of Vienna as a whole became hostile to him and refused to accept his teachings. It remained for Joseph Lister of London and Oliver Wendell Holmes of Massachusetts to gain recognition for the principles of surgical antisepsis.

Today, volatile organic chemicals may be the counterpart of infectious diseases in earlier times before there was any scientific understanding of their nature. Parents of today may be the counterparts of Semmelweis, recognizing the nature of childhood illnesses brought about by chemical exposures without questioning whether there is scientific proof.

In closing, let us return to the question posed in the title of this work: *Who is looking after our kids?* We do not claim to have all the answers, but one thing could be said without the slightest reservation: Parents should be allowed a larger voice in matters concerning the care, health, and well-being of their children than usually granted to them in our present society.

References

1. Chester AC, Levine PH. Concurrent sick building syndrome and chronic fatigue syndrome: epidemic neuromy-asthenia revised. *Clin Infect Dis.* 1994;18 (suppl 1):843-848.

2. *Multiple Chemical Sensitivities*. Washington, DC. National Research Council National Academy Press. 1989.

3. *Biological Markers of Reproductive Toxicology*. Washington, DC .National Research Council. National Academy Press. 1992.

4. *Environmental Neurotoxicology*. Washington, DC.National Research Council. National Academy Press. 1992.

5. *Pesticides in Diets of Infants and Children*. Washington, DC. National Research Council. National Academy Press.

APPENDIX II

Contaminated school buildings
by Doris Rapp, MD,
Pediatric Allergist, Buffalo, NY

From her presentation to the American Academy of Environmental Medicine in Virginia Beach, Virginia, 1994.

Wherever man goes, the earth hurts. (Indian saying)

Many children and teachers are being made ill by school buildings due to a combination of factors. The "sick building syndrome" may be due to chemicals, mold, dust, dust mites, bacteria, viruses, increased carbon dioxide levels and poor ventilation.

Clues that the child is made ill by the school environment:

Symptoms worsen during the day and lessen hours after the child returns home.

Symptoms worsen as the week goes on and lessen during weekends.

Symptoms lessen during vacations.

The "spreading phenomenon," in which there is increasing sensitivity to chemicals.

School locations of special problems:

Lavatories (disinfectants, deodorants)

Cafeterias (pesticides, allergic food reactions)

Basements (damp and moldy)

Gyms

Pools (chlorine reactions)

Chemistry and biology labs (chemicals)

School desks
(formaldehyde from particle boards, varnishes)

School buses (exhaust fumes)

Damp and musty classrooms (mold)

Ventilation systems (if contaminated, may permeate many areas of schools)

Art classes
(volatile chemicals, lead from art paint)

Crowded classrooms with poor ventilation (high levels of viruses and bacteria)

Pollen from outdoor air

Poor ventilation with outdoor air
(increased levels of carbon dioxide)

How to pinpoint the problem:

What were the conditions when symptoms or illness commenced? Observe the child before and after going into various rooms or locations of the school. Observe and record before and after reactions of the "big five:"

How did the child look before and after going in and out of rooms?

How did the child feel?

How did the child act, write, and draw? (Have child write and draw.)

Check pulse before and after.

Check breathing (peak flow meters available from our office).

For best documentation, take a video camera into the school.

Does the child come out of a room or location with red ears and red cheeks, with difficulty breathing, with behavioral changes, fatigue, and increased clumsiness?

Document with a video camera.

How does one document that there is a sick building?

Have an expert in heating and ventilation come in and examine the building.

Check the air for particles (dust, mold, pollen).

Check carbon dioxide levels (outdoor air 350 ppm — good indoor air 400 ppm—with levels of 1,000 ppm or 2,000 ppm, it becomes difficult to function).

Check for chemicals in the air.

What to check for:

Check for dust (dust mites).

Check for mold in damp and musty locations.

Carbon dioxide levels.

Check to see if pesticides and herbicides have been used. If they are used, encourage integrated pest management, a system of pest management without the use of chemicals. It is both more effective and less expensive. A number of school districts in the US and Canada are adopting these methods.

Check for new carpets, commonly sources of toxic chemical outgassings.

Check ventilation systems. Check ventilation filters to see if they are clean.

In crowded rooms with poor ventilation, check virus and bacteria levels.

Check furniture for chemical odors (formaldehyde, varnishes).

Check for radon, lead from old paint, asbestos.

Check for electromagnetic pollution (heavy wiring near a classroom).

Carbonless paper (source of formaldehyde)

Copying machines

Art supplies (glues, lead from art paint)

Medical tests for the child:

"Sick building blood panel" - a blood test available from laboratories that tests immune blood cells, antibodies against chemicals and smooth muscles in the body. Formaldehyde and trimellitic anhydride antibodies may be the most useful, as they tend to remain elevated for prolonged periods after chemical exposures. Positive trimellitic anhydride antibodies were found in 90% of patients with multiple chemical sensitivities. If TMA IgM antibodies are more than 1:8, it indicates current exposure. If TMA IgG antibodies are more than 1:8, it reflects previous exposure.

Blood levels for volatile organic compounds (AccuChem Laboratories, Richardson, TX)

SPECT Scan test of the brain.

Radioactive glucose is injected into the patient, which is taken up by the brain and photographed by scintigraphy. 100% abnormality was found in patients with multiple chemical sensitivity, who showed irregular and decreased uptake of radioactive glucose by the brain.

If possible, schedule tests for Fridays, because chemicals tend to accumulate during the week. Document the testing with a video camera.

Nerve conduction and muscle tests.

Provocation and neutralization tests for suspected chemicals (done in doctor's office).

Check formaldehyde with formic acid blood test.

Examples of the health hazards of sick buildings and their furnishings:

In a study, an 8 by 10 inch piece of a carpet one-year-old was placed next to a cage of mice. A fan was placed near the carpet, gently blowing air over the carpet into the cage of mice. After three hours, one mouse died!

Another example: a few years ago the Environmental Protection Agency (EPA) completed a new building, supposed to be the latest in modernization, in Washington, DC, as their headquarters. There was a problem, however, with the building. Shortly after occupancy, a large proportion of employees became ill. The source was traced to fugitive chemical out-gassings from carpets together with a defect in the ventilation system. The primary chemical offender was phenylcyclohexane (4-PCH) emitting from the latex backing of the carpets. Some time later the EPA did remove the carpets at millions of dollars expense. However, the EPA did not think there was enough evidence to warn the public.

How to correct a sick building:

Clean up dust and mold.

Air cleaners in classrooms.

Replace pesticides with integrated pest management: better and less expensive.

Use nontoxic cleaning solutions.

Do renovation such as indoor painting during summertime, so that chemicals will be largely dissipated before children return to school.

Check the ventilation system - don't rush into this - if chemicals are used to clean the system, they may be toxic and carried throughout the building.

Linoleum or wood floors are much easier to keep clean.

Linoleum is cheaper than carpets.

Where petrochemical fuels (oil, gas, kerosene) are used, check for leaks into indoor air.

Many other things could be mentioned, but those listed above are the most common sources of health problems.

How to treat children with health problems from sick buildings

Exercise

Saunas

Massage

Organic foods

Air purifiers in classrooms

Cotton clothes

Nutrient supplements including a multiple vitamin, multiple minerals, extra vitamin C, extra calcium and magnesium, essential fatty acids (Omega-3 and

Omega-6 oils), glutathione and taurine (necessary for body detoxification, valuable against inflammation).

Lactobacillus acidophilus and *bifidis*, to restore normal (healthy) intestinal flora when antibiotics have been used.

A small amount of bicarbonate (commercial Alka Seltzer Gold®) may be used several times daily to neutralize allergic or chemical reactions.

The yeast syndrome may be treated by physicians with Nystatin® or other agents.

Allergy extracts by physicians.

Pure drinking water (either spring water in glass bottles or a water purification device attached to the kitchen sink for drinking and cooking).

Some are successfully using homeopathic medications (less expensive).

Laboratory results with chemically injured children :

100% abnormal SPECT Scans; TMA antibodies elevated in 50%; 62% reacted to school air in provocation testing; 50% had immunologic changes in T and B cells. In general, the T-helper cells went down and the T-suppressor cells went up (the pattern generally seen in autoimmune diseases).

We are appreciative of Dr. Rapp for her diligent research and permission to use the above information.

APPENDIX III
Preconception care interview forms

For the prospective mother and father:

You are the very best source of information about your health, your body, your lifestyle and history. Please take some quiet time to thoughtfully answer the following questions so that our team of professionals can begin to construct a detailed profile of you, and your partner. This data, together with additional information obtained through interview and examination, will be used to develop a detailed and extremely personalized plan to optimize the wellness of your family while anticipating conception.

The information you give us is held in strictest confidence. You, of course, have complete access to your files at any time. Thank you for your cooperation.

(PLEASE PRINT)

Name: _____ Physician: _____
      Last   First
Address: _____ Address: _____
         Street   Street
_____ _____
City   State   Zipcode   City   State   Zipcode

Home Phone: ____-____-_____   Phone: ____-____-_____
Work Phone: ____-____-_____

Preconception Care Clinician: _____
Date of initial consultation: ____/____/____

Age_____
Date of Birth ____/____/____
Height ____ft. ____in.
Current weight _____
Heaviest weight _____   Date: from_____ to_____
Least weight _____   Date: from_____ to_____

Ethnic origin _____

OCCUPATIONAL HISTORY
Present Work _____

Previous Work History _____
_____
_____

Were you ever employed in an area with identified or suspected environmental hazards? _____

ETHNIC BACKGROUND
Father _____ Mother _____
Paternal Grandfather _____ Maternal Grandfather _____
Paternal Grandmother _____ Maternal Grandmother _____

157

For the prospective mother and father:

State whether there is any family history of heart disease, thyroid disease, diabetes, cancer, arthritis, neuro-muscular disease, birth defects or any other disease not listed above. _____

MEDICAL HISTORY
Please detail any present illness. Give dates when illness began and describe the time of day, duration and changes in the illness(s) over time. Is the illness connected to events such as eating, exercise etc.? What treatment have you received? Who treated you?

_____
_____
_____
_____
_____

Please detail any present complaints not connected to a medical diagnosis, such as "occasional tension headaches" or "severe indigestion". How frequently do these occur and do they seem to be connected to an event? Has medical or other professional help, such as chiropractic, a druggist or a friend been sought?

_____
_____
_____
_____
_____

Have you ever been treated for or had any of the following conditions?

1	Acne_____		35	Halitosis _____
2	Anorexia_____		36	Hayfever_____
3	Asthma_____		37	Headaches/migraines_____
4	Back Pain_____		38	Herpes_____
5	Bleeding Gums_____		39	High Blood Pressure_____
6	Bloating_____		40	High Raised Palate_____
7	Bloodshot Eyes_____		41	Hives_____
8	Body Odor (severe)_____		42	Hostility (no cause)_____
9	Bowel Cramps_____		43	Hyperactivity_____
10	Brittle Nails_____		44	Insomnia_____
11	Bruising_____		45	Irritable Bowel_____
12	Bulimia_____		46	Joint Pain_____
13	Burning Feet_____		47	Kidney Disorders_____
14	Cataracts_____		48	Memory Loss_____
15	Coeliac Disease_____		49	Mononucleosis_____

For the prospective mother and father:

```
16  Cold Feet_____      50  Mouth Ulcers_____
17  Cold Hands_____      51  Multiple Sclerosis_____
18  Constipation_____      52  Nervousness_____
19  Cystitis_____      53  Palpitations_____
20  Dandruff_____      54  Panic Attacks_____
21  Dental Decay_____      55  PMS_____
22  Depression_____      56  Rheumatoid Arthritis_____
23  Diabetes_____      57  Sciatica/Lumbago_____
24  Diarrhea_____      58  Sensitivity to noise_____
25  Dizzy Spells_____      59  Skin Disorders_____
26  Dyslexia_____      60  Stretch Marks_____
27  Ear Infections_____      61  Sweating (heavy)_____
28  Eczema_____      62  Swollen Feet_____
29  Enlarged Glands_____      63  Tinnitus_____
30  Epstein-Barr_____      64  Tuberculosis_____
31  Epilepsy_____      65  Urticaria_____
32  Fatigue/Lethargy_____      66  Varicose Veins_____
33  Frequent Urination_____      67  Weight Problems_____
34  Hair Loss_____      68  White Spots on Nails_____
```

Medications taken over the past year:
    Prescription:_____
    Over the counter_____

Have you ever had a problem in any of the following areas?

Head - eyes, ears, nose, sinuses _____

Neck and Throat_____

Breast_____
Cardiovascular_____
Respiratory_____

Endocrine - the function of any gland_____

Immune_____

Blood Problems - anemia, hemophilia etc._____

Lymphatics_____

Gastrointestinal_____

Urinary_____

Musculoskeletal_____

Neurologic_____

Psychiatric_____

For the prospective mother:

Did any of your babies weigh less than 5 lbs. at birth_____
more than 10 lbs. at birth_____

FAMILY PLANNING

Current method_____ For how long_____

Previous method/s_____

Problems with present of previous methods_____

Date of last pelvic exam_____ Pap smear_____
History of pelvic inflammatory disease_____
  Endometriosis_____
  Candida albicans_____
  Chlamydia_____
  Discharge_____Describe_____
  Pain on urinating_____
  Gonorrhea_____
  Herpes_____
  Mycoplasmas_____
  Mumps_____
  Non-specific Urethritis_____
  Thrust_____
  Streptococci_____
  Strapylococci_____
  Breast Disease, Benign_____
  Breast Disease, Cancer_____
  Cervicitis, Erosion_____
  Cervicitis, Positive Smear_____
  Ovarian Cysts_____
  Blocked Fallopian Tubes_____
  Fibroid Tumors_____
  Any other problems_____

ENVIRONMENTAL HISTORY

Occupational Environment (indicate length of employment)
  Mechanic_____   Lawn Care Specialist_____
  Printer _____   Electrician_____
  Lab Technician_____ Beauty Technician_____
  Painter_____   Other (describe)_____
  Factory Worker_____
  Chemist_____
  Exterminator_____

For the prospective mother:

REPRODUCTIVE HISTORY

Age of menarche (beginning of menstruation)_____
Date of first day of your last period_____
Number of days in cycle?_____
Are cycles regular?_____ Every_____days
Character of flow: Amount Copious (steady and enough)_____
                               Heavy (fast and too much)_____
                               Moderate_____
                               Light_____
                               Spotty_____
Does the flow change dramatically during the period?_____
Describe the change, and related timing_____

Are periods painful?_____
    Just before onset?_____
    During period?_____
    Irregularly?_____

Describe any premenstrual discomfort_____

Have you ever bled between periods?_____
Missed a period totally?_____
Been a week or more "late" in your cycle?_____

Have you ever been pregnant?------------ How many times?_____
Number of live births_____ Stillbirths_____
Number of abortions, elective of spontaneous_____

Complications of pregnancy:
    Early nausea lasting more than 8-12 weeks_____
    Spotting during pregnancy_____ When_____
    High blood pressure_____ Swelling of hands and feet____
    High blood sugar_____ Cardiac problems_____
    Other_____

Complications of labor and delivery:
    Prolonged _____ or very short (less than 3 hours)_____
    Excessive bleeding during labor_____

Normal vaginal delivery_____ Forceps Delivery_____
Breech delivery_____
Were pregnancies carried to term?_____

For the prospective father:

FAMILY PLANNING

Current method_____ For how long_____

Previous method/s_____

Problems with present of previous methods_____

Date of last pelvic exam_____ Pap smear_____
History of pelvic inflammatory disease_____
  Candida albicans_____
  Chlamydia_____
  Pain on urinating_____
  Gonorrhea_____
  Herpes_____
  Mycoplasmas_____
  Mumps_____
  Non-specific Urethritis_____
  Thrust_____
  Streptococci_____
  Strapylococci_____
  Undescended testicle_____
  Have you ever has a sperm test?_____
  Antibodies to sperm_____
  Low sperm count_____
  Poor sperm motility_____
  Malformed sperm_____
  Any other problems_____

Have you ever had children before?_____(Y/N) How Many?____

ENVIRONMENTAL HISTORY

Occupational Environment (indicate length of employment)
  Mechanic_____   Lawn Care Specialist_____
  Printer _____   Electrician_____
  Lab Technician_____ Beauty Technician_____
  Painter_____   Other (describe)_____
   Factory Worker_____
  Chemist_____
  Exterminator_____

For the prospective mother and father:

Have you ever been treated for:
Venereal Disease (Y/N)_____
Urinary Tract INfection (Y/N)_____
Please detail when and type of treatment:_____

Home Environment (indicate all that apply)

Have you done any recent renovations to your home or helped anyone renovate their home or work place?_____

    Painting_____
    Varnishing_____
    Paneling_____
    Insulating_____
    Wall-to-wall carpeting_____
    Other (please explain)_____

Materials (older homes)
    Plaster Walls_____
    Lead Plumbing_____
    Copper Plumbing_____
    Asbestos_____
    Iron Pipes_____
    Other (please explain)_____

Heating/Ventilation
    Forced hot air_____   Radiant_____
    Natural Gas_____   Oil_____
    Bottled Gas_____   Wood_____
    Electrical_____   Central Air Conditioning___
    Kerosene_____   Humidifier_____
    Room Air Conditioning_____   Dehumidifier_____
    In workplace (type)_____

Heavy Metal Pollution
    Algicides (swimming pool)_____   Lead Paint_____
    Aluminum (cooking)_____   Leaded Gasoline_____
    Aluminum (antiperspirants)_____   Mercury Fillings_____
    Antacids (brand)_____   Photocopiers_____
    Coffee Creamers_____   Selenium Shampoo_____
    Copper/Brass Jewelry_____   Soya Milk
    Foil Wrap_____   Tinned foods/drinks_____
    Grey Removers_____   Tuna Fish_____
    Henna dyes/rinses_____   Water Softeners_____

For the prospective mother and father:

```
Electrical Pollution
    Electric Blanket_____      Television/Computer_____
    Microwave oven_____      Personal Heater_____
    Tanning Salon_____      Overhead Power Lines_____
    Sun Lamps_____      Flourescent lights_____

General Pollution
    Fluoridation_____
    Pesticides_____      Mothballs/flakes_____
    Formaldehyde_____      Food Additives_____
    Gas Grill_____      Gas/electric stove_____
                                    Greenhouse foggers_____
    Herbicides_____
    Oven Cleaners_____      Insecticides_____
    Plastic food wrap_____      Termite Treatment_____
    Plastic food containers___      Third World Travel_____
    Plastic water bottles_____      Infra-red food heating
    Plastic storage bags for                       lamps_____
                       food_____  Hobbies_____
```

COMMON SOCIAL POISONS

Have you ever been treated for an addiction?_____

```
    Alcohol_____
    Anorexia_____
    Bulimia_____
    Coffee_____
    Drugs
        cocaine_____
        crack_____
        heroin_____
        marijuana_____
        speed_____
        valium_____
        other_____
    Sugar_____
    Tabacco_____  Brand_____  How long?_____
```

DIETARY STATUS (clinician will assess)
```
    Very Good_____
    Good_____
    Average_____
    Poor_____
    Comments_____
    _____
```

CLINICIAN WILL ASSESS (when necessary)
```
    Cytomegalovirus Status_____
    Rubella Status_____
    Toxoplasmosis_____
        Cat/s_____  How Long_____
```

INDEX

AIDS and the polio vaccine, 85
Allergies, food,
   testing for, 112-113
   treatment, 113
Antibiotics
   overuse of, 71
   immune impairment by, 71-72, 112
   overgrowth of pathogens from, 72-73
   alternatives to, 73-77
Antimony, 60
Aspartame, 27-30
Asthma, increasing incidence of, 4, 81
Autism Research Inst. 60, 63
Barnes, Belinda, preface
BHA, 23, 31
BHT, 23, 31
Birth defects in USA, 11
Blaylock, Russell, L, 27
Cadmium, 59
Chemical combinations,
   increasing toxicity of, 144
Chlordane, 19, 238-39
Clymer, R Swinburne, 117-118
DDT, 19, 38-39
Diamond, Marion, 123
Dioxin, 53
Egger, J, 30, 109-110
Estrogenic chemicals, 106-107
Feingold, Ben, 30
Finn, Ronald, 145
Fluorescent lights
   cool white, 51
   broad spectrum, 52
Fluoride,
   neurotoxicity of, 65

impaired memory from, 68
increased cancer from, 67
increased fracture from, 67
immune impairment from, 67-68
ineffectiveness of water fluoridation, 66-68
Food allergies,
   testing for, 112-113
   treatment for, 113
Food coloring, 30
Foods, organic,
   superior taste of, 17
   farming methods, 18
   superior in nutrients, 18-19
Formaldehyde, 42-43
Fudenberd, HH, 85-86,
Hyperactivity
   increasing incidence of, 5
   volatile organic compounds cause of, 34-35
Integrated pest management, 136-137
Lead, 53-54, 57-59
Low birth weights, incidence of in USA, 10
Lukesch, Monika, 121
Mercury, 59
Metal toxicity, management of, 61-63
Monosodium glutamate, (MSG), 27-30
Mortality, infant, in the USA, 10
Multiple chemical sensitivity,
   federal recognition of, 97-98
   causes, 98-99
   mechanisms, 99-100

diagnosis of, 100-101
treatment, 100-102
Nitrites, 31
Nitrates, 33
Organic foods,
  superior taste of, 17
  farming methods, 18
  superior in nutrients, 18-19
Organophosphate pesticides, 39-40, 135-136
Pangborn, J, 60, 63
Persian Gulf War Syndrome, 107
Pesticides
  DDT, 19, 38-39
  chlordane, 19, 38-39
  organophosphates, 39-40, 135-136
Plumbing, household, 53-54
Polychlorinated biphenyls, (PCBs), 53
Pre and Peri-Natal Psychology Association. of North America, 118
Preconception care,
  plan, 12-16
  history intake forms, 157-164
Rapp, Doris, 110-111, 149-157
Ritalin, 5
Scheibner, Vera, 82
Scholastic performance,
  improvement by diet, 23-24
Secretory IgA Immune system, 83, 111-112
Semmelweis, 123, 146
Shetler, Donald, 123-124
Sick building syndrome, 106
Smith, Lendon, 5
Solvents, 40-42
Stott, Dennis, 122

Sulfites, 31
SPECT brain scan, 100-101
Swanson, J,42
Vaccinations
  Tetanus, 84
  Measles, Mumps, Rubella (MMR), 84-85
  Polio, 85
  Measles, 87
  Measles vaccine, Crohn's disease and ulcerative colitis, 86-87
  chronic fatigue immune dysfunction and vaccines, 91-93
Verny, Thomas, 118-124
Violence, reduction of by diet, 24
Viral infections, increasing incidence of, 4, 81
Volatile organic compounds
  increased production of, 33-34
  neurotoxicity of, 33, 38
  causing hyperactivity, 34-35
  causing behavioral problems, 34-35, 42-44
  causing learning disabilities, 36-38, 42
Walker-Smith,J, 86, 87
Water pollution
  PCBs and dioxin, 53
  nitrates, 53
  lead, 53-54
  plastic pipes in plumbing systems, 54
  solvents and glues, 54
Whitaker, J, 75
Yiamouyiannis, John, 66-68

About the authors

Richard Piccola

Mr. Piccolo is the Executive Director of the Foresight-America Foundation for Preconception Care.

In 1990 he retired from his private business interests (health care strategic planning and systems design) and dedicated all of his efforts to designing a new paradigm in medicine that would be more responsible to the American public. Placing the patient's health and well-being first, the system would combine the best of allopathic, environmental and holistic medicine.

Harold E. Buttram, MD

Dr. Buttram is in private practice at Woodlands Medical Center in Quakertown, Pennsylvania in the fields of family practice and environmental medicine. Years of experience have convinced him that many of the physical and mental health problems among Americans today are in large measure the result of an increasingly toxic environment, children being the most vulnerable. For this reason, along with his medical practice, he regularly devotes time to various avenues of public education.

please photocopy this form

To:
1996 Foresight/America Foundation for Preconception Care
5724-B Clymer Rd.
Quakertown, Pennsylvania 18951

Please send me:
Our Toxic World: Who is looking after our kids?
A guide for parents to protect their children from toxic substances,
Harold Buttram, MD & Richard Piccola, MHA

I enclose a check or money order for $14.95 plus $3.00 shipping.

(This is your mailing label - please write clearly:)

Name:

Street Address:

City   State   Zip

Phone:

If ordering more than two books, please call for price: 215.529.9026